The Feel Good Fix

To my loving, supportive family and
my Feel Good community

Lavina Mehta MBE

The Feel Good Fix

Boost Energy, Improve Sleep and Move More Through Menopause and Beyond

PENGUIN LIFE

AN IMPRINT OF

PENGUIN BOOKS

PENGUIN LIFE

UK | USA | Canada | Ireland | Australia
India | New Zealand | South Africa

Penguin Life is part of the Penguin Random House group of companies
whose addresses can be found at global.penguinrandomhouse.com.

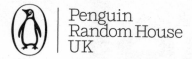

First published 2024
001

Copyright © Lavina Mehta MBE, 2024

The moral right of the author has been asserted

Set in 13.2/16pt Garamond MT Std
Typeset by Jouve (UK), Milton Keynes
Printed and bound in Great Britain by Clays Ltd, Elcograf S.p.A.

The authorized representative in the EEA is Penguin Random House Ireland,
Morrison Chambers, 32 Nassau Street, Dublin D02 YH68

A CIP catalogue record for this book is available from the British Library

ISBN: 978–0–241–66508–4

www.greenpenguin.co.uk

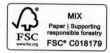

Penguin Random House is committed to a
sustainable future for our business, our readers
and our planet. This book is made from Forest
Stewardship Council® certified paper.

Contents

Feel Good Mentally

Feel Good for Life

Putting It into Action

Introduction

Are you trying to navigate midlife, perhaps battling with the common midlife weight gain, leading a busy life and maybe going through the hormonal roller coaster of perimenopause with its associated symptoms? Do you want to feel better and exercise more but feel demotivated, time poor, or unsure of what to do in the minefield of information out there? Are you worried about your long-term health and all the chronic diseases which are so common these days? Midlife is certainly the time for us to invest in our health, to help us age well and feel good today.

In this book, I'm going to share the Feel Good toolkit I use every day in my busy life. My hope is that this book will help you rethink the way you see exercise, by offering easy, quick, fun, innovative and effective workouts and bite-size exercise and life-style snacks to really make you feel good. To clarify, the term 'exercise snacking' is not to do with eating snacks – or exercising with your favourite food snack in hand! It is small amounts of activity, taken regularly throughout the day. This has been proven to have incredible health benefits – research has found that this method can be even more effective and beneficial than the single long workouts we struggle to fit in.

I understand the challenges of midlife because I'm going through it myself. Like you, I'm short on time, lacking motivation, tired from nights of broken sleep, juggling my children, work, family and home duties. Like most middle-aged women I feel trapped in the sandwich generation. I still have motherhood and home duties, as well as ageing parents. But I want to invest in myself too. I'm not perfect – that's why I really believe this flexible approach will work, whatever your schedule and lifestyle. All I know is that it's become the foundation to me feeling good, and it gives me the strength to cope with every aspect of my life.

I want to remove the common barriers to exercise of cost, time, motivation and even age and ability. I've had people up to the age of a hundred join my free virtual workouts, and I've found them so inspiring and motivating. Anything is better than nothing, and it's never too late to start. I want this book to provide accessible ideas, tips and solutions for all ages, to help you take that first step towards everyday habits that are sustainable in the long term.

I will show you that exercise can help give you more energy, more self-confidence, better sleep, more stable moods, better relationships, higher self-esteem. Menopause is not about becoming old, frail and tired, but about feeling stronger, happier and more able to face the challenges of midlife. Women are living longer, and I want us to understand the importance of investing in our health from midlife onwards. It will help our quality of life as we age.

Many of us don't meet the UK physical activity guidelines and, to be fair, finding the two and a half hours to exercise each week, plus two strength training sessions, recommended by the NHS can be a challenge. The WHO physical activity guidelines are even higher at 150–300 minutes of moderate-intensity aerobic physical activity, or at least 75–150 minutes of vigorous-intensity aerobic physical activity (or a combination) per week. That amount of time is so difficult for us all to find in midlife, with our families, work, kids and fast-paced lives. It's pretty daunting and intimidating for me! That's why I think it's life changing to know that exercising little and often is just as effective, if not *more* effective. Every minute counts, no amount of time is too small, and snacking on exercise also breaks up long periods of sitting, which is detrimental to our health.

This book provides 80+ easy and effective activity snacks to choose from, based on your ability, need and mood. They come with a variety of different focuses, intensity and lengths, are all free (unless you choose to treat yourself to some equipment) and can be done anywhere. You can pick 'n' mix them, depending on the time you have – and even 'stack' snacks to combine them. They may be small in terms of portion size, but they are every bit as effective as a longer, more traditional workout.

Despite the title, there is no magic fix, and no strict timetable or pressure or regimental plan. The 'fix' is satisfying your craving with the snacks, hacks, nibbles and tips, depending on how you're feeling and how much time you have. Giving you a satisfying fix that your body and mind craves and needs in order to feel good.

The Feel Good Fix is practical, easy and flexible enough to work around you and your lifestyle. I hope you get your fix with the snacks in this book!

Your health in midlife is the biggest predictor of your health in later life

Midlife health and the menopause

Perimenopause and menopause are key biological phases that 51 per cent of the population will have to navigate. Up until recently, there was no understanding of what perimenopause really is, let alone an awareness of the more than forty associated symptoms, many of which have led women to leave the workplace and their relationships. I know how tough it is to navigate, and my own perimenopause has challenged my relationships, self-esteem and mental strength. I want you to know that you are not alone and that we can get through this together. The Feel Good toolkit in this book has been fundamental in helping me through my own challenging journey, and I've seen so many women use it and thrive too.

Exercise can provide a brilliant solution to menopause symptoms, whether alongside or without HRT, as well as adopting healthy eating and positive lifestyle changes. Not only will exercise help you manage your symptoms and improve your quality of life now, but it will help future-proof you and reduce your risk of developing chronic illnesses later in life, such as diabetes, osteoporosis, Alzheimer's and dementia, heart disease and cancers – all diseases which women have an increased chance of contracting in midlife. A 2020 study found that sticking to a healthy lifestyle, including exercising regularly, is associated with a longer life expectancy at the age of fifty, free of major diseases. It's the simple, small changes you make today that are going to have a big impact on your future health.

When I first realized I was experiencing the perimenopause, I was in my early forties. I had confused the symptoms with long Covid. After GP appointments, tests and watching TV presenter Davina McCall's documentary, it dawned on me that I'd entered perimenopause around three years earlier, from the age of forty. I went live on Instagram the next morning, no make-up, still very tearful. It was a raw, honest conversation about my feelings, and I received a hugely overwhelming response. As a South Asian woman, there is so much that is not discussed in my community, from pregnancy, to sex, periods, mental health and, of course, the menopause. Everything happens behind closed doors, and we don't want to put ourselves out there. I received so many private messages from women who felt at rock bottom, and it broke my heart to see so many women suffering.

From broken marriages, to women who had left their jobs and fallen out with their teenage kids, many felt depressed (and were on prescription antidepressants) and some no longer had the will to live. Data from the Office of National Statistics shows that 60 per cent of all divorce petitions are initiated by women in their forties, fifties and sixties – the ages when women are typically going through the perimenopause, the menopause, or are post-menopause. There are devastating reports of women who have contemplated or tragically resorted to taking their own lives. In October 2021, the *Independent* newspaper reported exclusive research based on a survey of 2,000 women aged forty-six to sixty in the UK, which found that nine out of ten women going through the menopausal transition experienced mental health problems. One in ten experienced thoughts of suicide. If you are struggling with this huge life change, you really are not alone, and there are many things that can help. Some of them are included in this book but there are also fantastic organizations that offer support of every kind. See page 370 for a selection of organizations that may provide the help you need.

I kicked off sharing my perimenopause journey publicly on social media, raw and unedited – talking about the symptoms I was experiencing and the steps I had started taking – to make sure I and other women no longer suffer needlessly. I am a patron of Menopause Mandate, and every day I see how necessary it is to help women understand what perimenopause is, especially in

South Asian communities like mine (many of whom still don't know what the word means). It is time for us all to start taking charge of our health.

I know how the exercise, mind and lifestyle snacks in this book have helped me get through some of my most debilitating peri-menopause symptoms – from anxiety to weight gain, brain fog, joint aches, sleep issues, mood swings, lack of motivation and low self-esteem – as well as my irregular menstrual cycle. That's why I really want to share my experiences with you and help you find the tools to Feel Good. As women we need to support one another, to know that we can get help and be in control. I want us to feel empowered to take charge and find solutions.

As the perimenopause can start ten years before your meno-pause, women as early as their late thirties often start to notice hormonal symptoms affecting their weight and exercise, such as insomnia, lack of energy and mood dips. There are more than forty documented, common symptoms, though this list seems to be growing as research and awareness increases. It's worth pointing out that it looks like one in four women will experience debilitating symptoms, but one in four will also experience no symptoms at all. Remember that everyone is different, and your journey is unique to you. My main advice is to keep a log of your symptoms, so that you can get the help you need.

Mental health

Many women, like me, experience mental health issues for the first time in their lives during perimenopause, at the very time when our coping skills and mental resilience seem depleted. Several of the symptoms of perimenopause could be grouped under the heading of 'emotional well-being', while others – such as muscle tension, headaches, bloating and skin issues – could be caused by stress. The psychological and emotional symptoms, which include problems with memory, mood swings, anxiety, depression, panic disorders and irritability, are frustrating to deal with, and can be harder to pinpoint to hormones. But they are very common during peri/menopause, and therefore important to highlight, especially as oestrogen levels dip, which can affect brain function and the production of feel-good chemicals.

I have made mental health and mind snacks a big focus in this book as part of a toolkit to help us manage stress, as most symptoms can be improved by calming our nervous system. Physical movement through exercise snacking goes hand in hand with these, to help us improve our mood and our emotional well-being.

Mood swings

The causes of mood swings in menopausal women are complex, although research has linked low mood to fluctuating hormones. Oestrogen plays a role in many brain functions, so falling levels during the perimenopause may affect psychological well-being in some women. It's important to understand this; just knowing that this is beyond your control can be helpful.

I have heard so many women, friends and clients complain of irrational anger during perimenopause. I myself have experienced out-of-character mood swings when there is no real cause for them. The hormonal roller coaster is real. Unfortunately, it can have an impact on everyone else around you too. I always feel terrible when the sudden outbursts of screaming have been directed at those I love the most. It's not always easy to keep a lid on emotions in my male-dominated house, with a blend of teenage and menopausal hormones in the air.

At this stage of life, many of us also experience other stresses, such as children leaving home, or caring for an elderly relative, which can increase our feelings of anxiety and depression. Women are more likely than men to develop an anxiety disorder, depression, headaches, migraines and even some types of brain tumours. That's why we must find ways to help us navigate the challenges of midlife.

As oestrogen declines, serotonin production and receptors are affected, but exercise is one of the best ways to combat these changes, as it increases hormones like serotonin, norepinephrine and dopamine, to help improve mood and reduce depression. Endorphins – the 'feel good' sensation – are released immediately after exercise; like the 'runner's high', it's a euphoric state that typically involves elated, contented feelings and a general sense of well-being. This natural hormonal cocktail is like a calming, energizing pick-me-up shot that can power you through the remainder of your day. Even a single exercise snack can have cathartic effects on your brain.

Anxiety

Anxiety is a common symptom of the menopause transition, with one survey showing that over half of the women interviewed (aged forty-five to sixty-five and transitioning through the menopause) experienced mood changes. It can make you feel fearful or tense, unable to cope, overwhelmed – and it can hit you suddenly or creep up on you slowly.

Exercise can work wonders for anxiety in multiple ways – it increases your sense of well-being, your self-worth, body confidence and feelings of happiness. Research has shown that exercise promotes the growth of neurons in the hippocampus (a deep part of the brain responsible for learning and memory), so people who exercise tend to be able to handle stress better. The hippocampus of a person who lives a sedentary lifestyle consists of untrained neurons, which are by nature easily excitable, and 'fire' easily when confronted with a minor stressor. This, in turn, can make situations, decisions and even thoughts appear more stressful, and make us feel more anxious than we should. So, through exercise, we can strengthen healthy neural connections in the hippocampus. The less we sit and the more we move, we effectively reprogram the brain – as it's so adaptable – to deal with stress more easily.

There is ample evidence that partaking in low- to moderate-intensity exercise on a weekly basis can help improve anxiety in middle-aged and older women. Studies have also found that those who exercised regularly were less likely to be depressed and experienced fewer symptoms than those who did not exercise often.

Giving ourselves the headspace to complete tasks and juggle life's demands is easier said than done at times, and we tend not to put ourselves first. But finding time for our own self-care is so important. The mind snacks in this book, especially the breath snacks, can be a fabulous tool in helping you reduce your anxiety by helping to reset your nervous system in a matter of minutes.

Brain fog

Have you ever struggled to remember things, names of people or events from your past, find it hard to concentrate, or have experienced brain fog? You may, at times, have found yourself standing in a room wondering why on earth you are there, or started a sentence and forgotten what it was that you needed to say? Although 'brain fog' isn't an actual medical condition, it's a term that describes a range of symptoms which affect your ability to think. You may feel confused, forgetful or disorganized, or find it hard to focus or put your thoughts into words. I certainly have, and often call it 'cotton wool brain'.

You are not alone in experiencing menopause brain! Over 60 per cent of women report cognitive difficulties during their menopause transition, and for nearly two-thirds of women menopause comes with an undesirable change in memory. A lot of women, like me, worry that these are early signs of dementia. But if these problems with brain function coincide with changes in hormone levels, they are far more likely to be signs of menopause.

Nevertheless, I did feel like I was going mad. From the countless times my boys and husband would say, 'We've already told you!' and, 'Mum, how have you forgotten this?!' to going to important work events and struggling to recall people's names. Any symptoms related to menopause, including the effects on brain function, have to be seen in the context of everything else that is going on in your life. My perimenopause started at the same time as embarking on a new career path, whilst also juggling home and family. Menopause often coincides with other significant life events, such as adult children leaving home, the arrival of grandchildren, the development of chronic diseases, including diabetes or heart disease, ageing parents requiring care, or planning for transition to retirement.

The good news is that exercise could be one tool to help you reduce brain fog. I know it has helped me so much. Exercise changes the brain in ways that help to protect memory and thinking skills. Aerobic exercise (cardio) and resistance (or strength) training help your brain to function more efficiently. Just as all body structures need good blood flow to function and repair, the brain similarly requires good blood flow to maintain optimal function. I personally find walking to be one of the best ways to banish brain fog – outdoors, and ideally in nature, for even more mental health benefits. It doesn't have to be a long walk, it can just be a walk snack (see page 207) for five minutes, but I find it always freshens and energizes the mind. There are lots of snacks in this book to choose from to boost your brain.

Weight gain

Let's talk about the menopause pot belly and the hot topic of weight gain. During midlife our bodies' response to exercise changes. Maintaining a healthy weight, which once may have been so easy to do, may not work any more, even though you're doing exactly what you used to do.

Around 70 per cent of women will gain weight during menopause. I have experienced this myself. I look back nostalgically at the photos that were taken of me when I first qualified as a personal trainer, lean and with a six-pack, just before perimenopause began! I instil the message to 'exercise for sanity, not vanity' but I know how it feels when your clothes don't fit properly any more, and how frustrating it feels when the weight suddenly appears, even though you haven't really changed that much with your nutrition or exercise routine. My belly is now soft and squidgy most days, and the bloating during my perimenopause has hit me hard. As a personal trainer I've learnt to respect how we view our own bodies – to others I may look exactly the same, but I feel the changes. I think people expect a personal trainer to look a certain way, which has some associated pressure, but I'm accepting my body's development and am ageing positively.

Why the gain in weight?

During menopause your oestrogen levels decrease. When that happens, you gain a tendency to accumulate fat, especially around the abdomen, and also to lose muscle mass. The result is the telltale belly and love handles. This happens because when your ovaries stop producing oestrogen, your body searches for it elsewhere, and the only other place it is generated is in the abdominal fat cells. Your body stores fat there in an effort to increase oestrogen levels. The fat cells – also called adipose tissue – are actually serving a helpful role as they're preserving and producing some oestrogen, which is essential in our bodies and good for our hormonal health. The gut is also affected by the hormonal changes in perimenopause, and bloating is a common symptom; you may have more gas, changes in your bowel movements, or slower digestion.

It is worth pointing out that low oestrogen can affect your ability to handle stress. If you're constantly in high stress mode, you will produce more cortisol and, most likely, become less sensitive to insulin, which means you're less able to lower your blood sugar levels after a meal. This can also lead to weight gain, especially in the belly area. Luckily, you can use the tips in this book, especially exercise and stress management, to help control the hormone cortisol and improve your insulin responses.

Menopot

The seemingly inevitable weight gain associated with peri/menopause, especially in the belly area, is often named the 'menopot'. Unfortunately, this new or expanded pot belly can develop even if you're on track with your nutrition and maintain a regular workout schedule, thanks to a number of factors unique to the menopause.

Weight around your middle is not only upsetting but can also increase health risks, including a greater chance of cardiovascular problems and metabolic disease. That's why women are at higher risk of heart disease and type 2 diabetes after midlife. Women tend to put on about 1–5 lbs each year in their fifties and sixties because of hormones plus muscle loss. Since muscle burns more calories than fat, this causes the metabolism to slow down. So, even if you're eating the same amount you always have, you're likely not burning the calories at the same rate as you once did. As you continue to lose muscle mass (unless you work on building it up) the problem can get worse, leading to faster weight gain. That's why it's key to do strength training.

You can read more about how and what to do in the Strength section that starts on page 61.

What we can do about it

It is quite common for women not to be exercising consistently, to be more sedentary, to be eating too much and too many processed foods, and not sleeping well. If you're in a heightened, stressed state, it's not ideal for your general well-being. Hence it's very important to start gaining control of your health. I hope the easy suggestions in this book help you to do this and to take some positive steps.

I want us to reframe the way we think about exercise, with a focus on long-term physical health, mental health and how we feel. We may have to start to come to terms with some weight gain, accept the changes that happen to our bodies as we age gracefully, and take some of the pressure off by not pursuing an overly lean body or unattainable six-pack (which would actually be detrimental to our physical and mental health).

Exercise for health and longevity. Use strength training to shift your focus from the weight on the scales to a more empowering measurement: the weight you can lift!

Unfortunately, menopause does mean that we store fat more easily and it's harder to lose it. But we also lose muscle, which is more metabolically active than fat, so we need to focus on building lean muscle mass. Improving our nutrition, plus self-care stress management techniques, alongside strength training, can all help. These are covered in this book, with plenty of choices and tips to help you feel good.

Women are massively underrepresented in all areas of research, especially studies of weight loss, and the research and subsequent advice are heavily biased towards men, though I'm sure more information on this will become available over time. I definitely don't recommend eating less and working out more in menopause. This will actually make the problem worse by overloading an already highly stressed body, with no time to apply any much-needed self-care, rest or recovery, which can lead to inflammation and further weight gain.

It's all about balance, nourishing yourself with my Feel Good methods; embracing, accepting and looking after yourself.

Sleep

Bad, broken or light sleep is something I've always struggled with since becoming a mum and living in a busy extended family, with nine of us under one roof, when I got married. Lack of sleep is a form of torture. My experiences, combined with perimenopause, just add to the anxiety I have most nights around whether I'll be getting a good night's sleep.

Many women who have always enjoyed a good sleep routine suddenly start experiencing insomnia or broken sleep in midlife. They put it down to stress, family or work issues, and the juggling act that comes at this stage of life. But we now know that sleep is intimately connected to our hormones as they start changing. Insomnia is a symptom of menopause reported by up to 40 per cent of women. When progesterone levels start declining, and as we age, our melatonin production is affected, which is the sleep-signalling hormone that helps us fall and stay asleep. As our sleep is affected, our mood, energy, performance, concentration, hunger and appetite levels, and even our motivation to exercise, are all affected. It often becomes a vicious circle, when we start to obsess and worry before bed.

Exercise and sleep are linked; each is essential for the other. Head over to the detailed section on sleep starting on page 313 for more information and my top tips.

Hot flushes

As oestrogen declines in perimenopause, this could affect thermo-regulation, causing an increase in core body temperature and hot flushes. Hot flushes can happen at any time of day or night. Night-time hot flushes may wake you up, further affecting your quality of sleep. As many as 80 per cent of women will experience hot flushes and night sweats during the menopause transition and beyond, but more research is still required into the exact causes.

The last thing you probably want to think about when you're having hot flushes is making yourself even hotter by working out. But early studies are showing that a regular, moderately intensive workout (yes, that means getting a bit hot and sweaty) may actually help reduce hot flushes (as well as provide a host of other benefits).

In fact, building muscle through lifting weights and strength training could also help lower the frequency and impact of flushes. Data from the Study of Women's Health Across the Nation (SWAN) found that maintaining higher levels of lean body mass (aka muscle) during the menopause transition may protect against the development of disruptive menopausal symptoms such as hot flushes and night sweats. Although there's no promise that you can avoid hot flushes altogether, I think it's very encourag-ing. You'll find lots of strength snacks in this book to help you get started.

One study using a simple breathing technique like the Mindful Minute 5.5 Breath Snack on page 273 has been shown to reduce hot flushes and calm the nervous system. It's such an easy snack, and one you can do anywhere, so it's definitely worth a try.

Joint pain

How many of you have experienced new niggly aches and pains once you hit perimenopause? It's often assumed that your joints can't take what they used to as you age, and so you view it as an inevitable part of getting older.

Oestrogen can reduce inflammation between joints, so when it fluctuates or decreases in perimenopause, many women can experience joint pain and stiffness. These symptoms may also be an indicator of reduced collagen and tissue production, resulting in a lack of support to the joints from reduced levels of cartilage and connective tissue.

I myself have naturally cut back on the amount of high-impact exercises in my daily routine (like burpees, jumping lunges, squat jumps etc.), which I used to be able to do in my thirties pain free! I have turned to snacking on HIIT, often doing low-impact versions of the exercises (which are still super effective) or for much shorter time periods (I'm talking seconds or minutes as opposed to the 30–60 minute HIIT classes I used to do in the gym). Personally, I have struggled with my knee for the last few years. I have thanked strengthening exercises like the Squat Snack on page 221 and the Lower Body Strength Snack on page 114 in helping me to target and build the muscles that support my knees. These snacks, combined with mobility snacks, stretch snacks and recovery snacks (like the Cold Water Snack on page 338) have thankfully reduced my knee flare-ups. When I do feel any pain, I focus on these exercises even more and they have enabled me to bounce back much faster. Strength snacks and balance snacks can also be beneficial as they help to strengthen the muscles and tissues surrounding the bones, which reduces the risk of falls and of sustaining long-term damage.

As we age it's quite common to experience osteopenia and osteoarthritis, combined with the menopausal symptoms of painful and stiff joints, all of which means you probably won't feel like exercising. But it's actually beneficial if you do, and exercise can help ease the pain. Exercise actually increases strength, makes moving easier, reduces joint pain and helps fight tiredness. That's why exercise snacking is so much more accessible and a great place to start. It doesn't have to be a long workout session; you can start off small, listen to your body and build up confidence.

Make sure you are eating a nutritious diet alongside exercising. It's worth checking your levels of key vitamins like Vitamin D, which can worsen joint pain if they are low. Magnesium is a great mineral to help reduce muscle aches and pains too, and it comes in spray form, but I also love having a soak in magnesium salts. Check out the self-care nibbles on page 269 for more ideas.

Exercise for Sanity, not Vanity®

I want to emphasize the mental health benefits of exercise, and I really want us to remove the focus on how we look. Instead, I want us to prioritize how exercise makes us *feel*. The snacks and tips in this book can be used to help us feel good and to thrive during the menopause and beyond.

Let's celebrate what our bodies can do rather than how we look. Becoming strong physically has made me stronger mentally too. Techniques like strength training have had a huge impact on my mind, and have made me more resilient, empowered and confident. Investing in my mental health through the concepts in this book has had a ripple effect on my relationships, my work and managing my perimenopause and has enabled me to tackle the challenges of midlife better. These techniques have kept me sane. I totally believe in strong body, strong mind.

The narrative around women needing to look a certain way and be smaller has meant many women have been striving for aesthetics rather than health goals. Aspiring to a six-pack is not very realistic, nor is it sustainable, and it can actually be detrimental in the long run and cause many women to quit exercising altogether. We need to reframe the way we look at fitness and health, focusing not just on what we can see but on the magic it does for us inside, on the benefits for our mental health and for our bones, brain, heart and long-term health as we age.

Diabetes and heart health

Diabetes hits women hard, especially at midlife. Menopause causes a sharp decrease in oestrogen levels in the body, leading to various changes that can affect bodyweight, fat distribution (like carrying more weight round the midriff), blood pressure and insulin sensitivity. These changes can raise your risk of type 2 diabetes, taking into account factors for age and ethnicity. The changes can also make managing existing diabetes more challenging.

I have many close family members and friends with diabetes, and it's particularly close to my heart as I lost my grandfather to it. South Asians are six times more likely to have type 2 diabetes, leading to higher risks of serious health complications, especially heart disease.

People with diabetes are encouraged to exercise regularly to promote better blood sugar control and to reduce the risk of cardiovascular diseases. As an ambassador for Diabetes UK, the important message and good news I want you to hear is that type 2 and pre-diabetes are largely preventable and even reversible through exercise, healthy eating and positive lifestyle changes.

A study published in the *British Journal of Sports Medicine* says that you may only need 11 minutes of exercise each day to live longer, because it lowers your risk of developing age-related health problems such as cardiovascular disease and type 2 diabetes. On the other hand, sedentary activity, which is any low-energy activity that involves sitting, reclining or lying, is linked with increased incidence of disease and early death. But 'exercise snacking' has also been shown to reduce blood sugar levels by up to 40 per cent, so every small amount counts.

Heart disease is the leading cause of death for women. Although we often focus on cardio/aerobic activity, less well known is the fact that muscle mass is extremely good for your heart. A 2021 study published in the *Journal of the American Heart Association* found that women with high levels of muscle mass are less likely to die from heart disease. In fact, women should prioritize building muscle mass over losing weight, to improve their cardiovascular health. Skeletal muscle (specifically musclin, a hormone-like messenger substance of the skeletal muscle), which is produced during exercise, protects your heart in a number of ways, including improving blood sugar management, boosting your metabolic health, as well as giving you the strength and energy to be more active and to stay fit.

Lifting weights also reduces the risk of type 2 diabetes through enhanced insulin sensitivity. This is because the muscles which are working use more glucose than the muscles which are resting. Muscle movement leads to greater sugar uptake by muscle cells and results in lower blood sugar levels. That's why strength training is of particular importance. The more lean muscle you have, the greater your storage area for mopping up excess sugar from your meals, and the more sensitive you become to insulin. Maintaining insulin sensitivity is important during the menopause transition and beyond, when we can become more insulin resistant. Since insulin resistance has been linked to excess weight gain during menopause, it can also help with body composition.

Health span, not lifespan

How long do you want to live? No matter what your answer is to the question, we can all agree on one thing, that we want to remain independent, healthy and free from disease for as long as possible. It's important to look at our health span, not just our lifespan. Lengthening our health span starts with thinking about how we can age well holistically, meaning prioritizing our physical health, mental health and daily lifestyle factors all in one (which is what this book aims to cover). It also means prioritizing ways to feel joy and connection, which can reduce stress and the risk of chronic health conditions. The snacks in this book are not necessarily going to give you a bikini body, but they will help you stay healthier for longer.

Dr Peter Attia is an expert in longevity and believes in the quality of the life we are living. He says longevity is a function of lifespan and health span. Lifespan is the number of years you live, and health span is a measure of how well, not necessarily how long, you live. Most people want both! We need to focus more on our health span – the number of years we live in good health – rather than just counting our lifespan, the number of years we're alive. Our objective should be to die 'with' disease, not 'of' disease, and a huge part of Dr Attia's philosophy is about aggressively taking action to delay the onset of common diseases. He believes that when it comes to longevity, exercise is the most important area to focus on. How you move defines how you live. He says it's not about exercising more, especially as we get older. It's about exercising intentionally.

Muscle is key for longevity

Muscle mass is vital to longevity, independence and strength as we age. Research from the National Institute on Aging explains that 'a big culprit for losing our physical abilities as we grow older is the age-related loss of muscle mass and strength . . . in addition to making everyday tasks difficult, mobility limitations are also linked to higher rates of falls, chronic disease, nursing home admission, and mortality.' Dr Gabrielle Lyon is a pioneer in this area and emphasizes that we should be 'focusing on building muscles rather than losing fat. Muscle will help you build your body armour to protect you throughout life.' We will then have more protection against type 2 diabetes and heart disease (as the more muscle mass we have, the better our glucose control and insulin sensitivity.) When we go through menopause, our sex hormones decrease, our insulin resistance increases, our blood flow decreases, and our protein signalling decreases (to combat this, 'women have to focus on their protein intake'). Muscle mass will help with our hormonal balance, boosting our mental clarity, elevating our mood' and helping us to feel good.

As we age, our muscles naturally lose mass, strength and the ability to grow, putting us at higher risk of developing many chronic diseases such as type 2 diabetes, high blood pressure, as well as obesity, frailty, and the resultant loss of freedom. Muscles help us control our glucose levels (which is the sugar in our blood stream). Our muscles use and mop up this glucose as fuel. Building muscles improves our insulin sensitivity (which is our ability to lower our blood sugar level after a meal), helping us to combat type 2 diabetes (look back at the section on 'Diabetes and heart health' on page 20).

Building muscles can actually help you live longer. Studies show that people who have more muscle mass are at a lower risk of death from all causes. Muscle mass is one of the strongest predictors of longevity, even more significant than weight or BMI. So it's essential for us to build muscle.

You're never too old to lift weights. Strength training not only builds muscle mass but can also work wonders in boosting your brain, heart, bones and mental health (more on this later). If nothing else, I hope this book gets you into strength training. This isn't about bulking up, this is about building longevity.

My goal is to encourage more women to take up strength training, to build muscle and prevent osteoporosis, as part of a balanced training programme alongside cardio activities such as walking, plus incorporating the holistic principles of breath, stretch and mobility. I know how crucial strength training is for women during the peri/menopause and for promoting longevity. I'm so glad that I have had all this experience training others – and myself – before I even started my own perimenopause journey. I have proved that my Feel Good method really works!

Research shows that exercising for as little as 11 minutes could prevent:

- 1 in 10 premature deaths
- 1 in 20 cases of cardiovascular disease
- Nearly 1 in 30 cases of cancer.

Isn't that amazing? Just by doing half the NHS's recommended amount, which equates to only 11 minutes per day.

Beyond menopause

The way we think about fitness and health needs to change in midlife and can be a vital tool in helping us cope with the symptoms of peri/menopause, but my Feel Good prescription doesn't stop there. It is my belief that it's never too late to start making small changes to improve our health. So I have researched and created specially designed chair-based exercises that I even persuaded my quite reluctant and camera-shy then 73-year-old mother-in-law to join me in demonstrating on my Instagram and YouTube live videos.

One of my mottos in life is, 'It's never too late!' This has been confirmed by the thousands of post-menopausal women who have joined my Feel Good workouts, demonstrating the power of movement at any age and level of ability. So if you're older reading this (or buying this book for your mum or grandmother), there are no age limits, this book is for you too! I only became a personal trainer at the age of forty and started exercising consistently during my thirties. I've come to realize that it doesn't matter *when* you find what works for you. It just matters that you *start*.

Know that every minute counts. One study found that for those over the age of sixty-five, even a minute of exercise is beneficial to your health, so it's better to do something rather than nothing! According to a Bath University study, adults can get stronger even with short bursts of exercise. The research found that doing two five-minute exercise snacks a day was enough to improve muscle mass and power in the over seventies. Studies have also confirmed the effectiveness of strength and resistance training in older adults with sarcopenia (age-related muscle loss). One study showed that a six-week squat exercise routine could improve hand grip strength and knee extensor strength in older women with sarcopenia. Research clearly demonstrates that strength-training exercises have the ability to combat weakness and frailty and their debilitating consequences. Muscle is the most plastic tissue we have and if we give it a stimulus, it responds quickly. We can increase muscle mass enormously – so with strength exercises in particular, it's really never too late to start.

This backs up what I've seen in my own workouts, and it echoes the countless feedback I've received over the years from people reducing their osteoarthritis, reversing type 2 diabetes, lowering cholesterol and blood pressure, gaining strength and maintaining their independence. I saw the increase in bone density with my own mother-in-law when she had a fall in the driveway. The doctor was shocked when the X-ray revealed no broken bones, and she said she'd been doing strength training with her daughter-in-law for two years. I have had a lovely lady in her seventies join me live every week, and even a fall which fractured her shoulder has not stopped her from taking part and doing some of the moves with a single arm – she says the strength my workouts have provided has helped her recovery and boosted her mental strength.

Alzheimer's and dementia

I lost my grandmother to Alzheimer's. I watched her deteriorate and struggle for the last decade of her life, and I am now an ambassador for the Alzheimer's Society charity.

Did you know that the early onset of dementia can start in your thirties or forties? I highlight this as much as I can – and I hope it's got your attention here. Dementia starts before you get symptoms, and you can take preventive action now.

Women have a greater risk of developing dementia during their lifetime. In fact, two-thirds of people with Alzheimer's disease (the most common type of dementia) are women, so for every man living with Alzheimer's there are two women. Although it had been thought that the main reason was because women live longer than men – and old age is the biggest risk factor for this disease – in fact, in most industrialized countries the difference in life expectancy is only four years.

A whole body of diverse recent research has shown that hormones likely play a major role in determining dementia risk, especially in menopause as oestrogen declines, triggering Alzheimer's in some women. These hormones are just as important for our brain health as they are for our reproductive health. The good news is that exercise can help to delay the onset of dementia.

Exercise your brain

Brain health must be seen as a vital part of well-being, alongside our physical health. Your brain is flesh, and it likes exercise. It needs blood flow, and what's good for your heart is good for your brain. Train it, exercise it, grow it. Like any muscle, if you don't use it you'll lose it!

The research is now showing that the benefits of exercise on brain health might be even more pronounced in women. Your level of fitness in midlife is strongly correlated with your brain health later on in life. Exercise reduces the risk of dementia by increasing brain-derived neurotrophic factor (BDNF), which is an essential protein compound (rather like a miracle growth fertilizer) essential for increasing neuroplasticity, maintaining healthy neurons and creating new ones. That's correct – it increases existing brain cells and builds new brain cells! When we exercise, the brain bathes itself in BDNF – and there's no trip to the pharmacy required. The best thing is that this drug is free – the prescription is simply to move more!

If you are physically active and fit in midlife, you have a 30 per cent lower risk of dementia later in life, compared to a middle-aged woman who is sedentary and not working out regularly.

Neuroscientist Wendy Suzuki says, 'The more you're working out, the bigger and stronger your hippocampus and prefrontal cortex gets. This is important because the prefrontal cortex and the hippocampus are the two areas that are most susceptible to neurodegenerative diseases and normal cognitive decline in ageing.' Hence why I truly believe in the power of snacking on bite-size exercise throughout the day.

My mission to get Asians fit

For South Asians menopause is still a taboo subject and one that needs more education and awareness. Many people don't realize that South Asian women are more likely to go through menopause five or six years earlier than the average white female. It's such an underexplored area, the research to date lacks representation, and we stick to the oft-quoted 'average age of fifty-one' without questioning it, when it could be closer to forty-five or forty-six for some women. As perimenopause can start up to ten years before this, South Asian women in their mid-thirties (soon after childbirth) need to be aware and invest in their health. There's no question in my mind that more work needs to be done on the subject to make the data more inclusive for all populations. What makes the problem more complex is that, whatever your background, everyone's journey is different.

Studies have shown that South Asians are likely to be less physically active than the average population in England, with only 55 per cent of South Asians hitting the recommended 150 minutes of physical activity per week. In addition, South Asians in the UK are six times more likely to have diabetes than the white population, and they have a two-fold increase in the risk of heart disease. These statistics really concerned me. With similar issues being observed globally, I began my mission to shake up the Asian community. I wanted to educate them and start changing their habits with my free tips, workouts and advice about exercise and healthy eating.

I was born in London but my parents are Indian (Gujarati) and came to the UK in the 1960s after being raised in Mombasa in Kenya. There is a history of diabetes and heart attacks in my own family, as is the case in most South Asian families. As a mum to three boys, it was really distressing to see how my parents' generation – and first-generation South Asians in Britain in general – were 'at risk' communities. It demonstrated the urgent need to develop interventions to engage this disproportionately affected community. Hence I began my mission to change things.

My goal is to raise awareness and spread the message that we can reduce the risks of prevalent chronic illnesses (such as type 2 diabetes, Alzheimer's, dementia, osteoporosis and heart disease) through physical activity and exercise, and by maintaining a healthy weight and eating well. I understand the culture, the social barriers and the taboos surrounding topics such as exercise. I want to break down these barriers by working with, rather than against, the cultural norms, through sharing my own experiences and showing both the older and younger generations how to make long-term lifestyle changes. I want to help as many people as possible globally.

Exercise snacking

So let me tell you properly about the healthiest type of snacking there is . . . *exercise snacking*.

It's free, accessible, easy and quick to build into your everyday life. Rather than doing 30–60 minutes of exercise all in one agonizing go, you can break your session into smaller bite-size snacks throughout the day. Studies have shown that these snacks have the same, if not even greater, health benefits. I think this is life changing. And I want this to change your life too! Think of exercise snacks as a treat for your body and mind.

Better for your health

The research behind exercise snacking shows that doing exercise in small bite-size chunks can be an easier way to get your exercise and may even help you burn more calories, lose more weight, and improve your blood glucose levels and blood pressure, to a greater degree than working out in larger chunks.

Professor Marie Murphy of Ulster University and Edinburgh University's research teams found that short bouts of exercise that add up to the same total amount are just as good as if not better for you than one long concentrated thirty-minute workout. I spoke to her and confirmed that it may even be more effective at improving blood glucose, reducing blood pressure and improving metabolic health than longer workouts. This is because when we stop exercising, our increased metabolism keeps going a little, while we recover, and exercise snacking increases the number of times we increase or boost our metabolism. So by doing exercise multiple times, we get multiple benefits. This builds up over a day or a week and leads to us using more energy. It is also possible that exercise snacking allows us to reach higher levels of intensity by working hard then taking a rest before the next bout. There is even some evidence that body mass and LDL cholesterol levels (which can increase the risk of heart attack and stroke) were further improved by exercise snacking.

Let's recap this, as it amazes me to this day: Professor Murphy's study shows no difference between exercise completed all in one go versus movement accumulated throughout the day, on our fitness levels, insulin and glucose levels. And other studies show that these exercise snacks, all added up, may even be better for improving blood pressure, bodyweight and cholesterol.

No cost

Exercise doesn't have to be difficult or cost anything. We don't always have the time, motivation or energy for a sixty-minute workout, and we don't need that.

You don't need an expensive gym membership or fancy equipment, you can work out from home with food tins and plastic bottles filled with water. If the 2020 Covid pandemic has taught us anything, it might be that home workouts really are effective.

Easier to fit into our busy lives

Most importantly, it's easy to fit into your life, particularly if you're new to exercise or if you want to build more movement into your day but you don't have much time.

Lack of time is the most common barrier and the reason most

frequently cited when it comes to not exercising. I also had an interesting chat with Professor Murphy about time and how she feels that it's actually a false or perceived barrier. How do you spend your time? When it came to preparing for my TED talk, I saw a study that showed the average time spent on social media is 2.5 hours a day. That's exactly what the UK exercise guidelines have been asking for in a week! So, think about how you spend that finite time budget of twenty-four hours a day. How do you prioritize your time? The good news is that exercise snacking gets rid of one of the excuses.

Takes your mind off your troubles

Professor Murphy also mentioned the mental health benefits, which I'm very passionate about. She said, 'Small bouts of exercise are great at taking your mind off what you're doing now and switching your attentional focus.' What a great tool this can be, especially for women who are juggling so many things all the time!

Snack on strength training

Another important thing to think about when choosing your snacks is how you spend this time exercising. I was thrilled to hear that Professor Murphy is as passionate about strength training as I am, and that's where we should be prioritizing our efforts – making sure it's an integral part of any exercise plan. Strength training is the most direct way to increase muscle mass and prevent its loss.

Her opinion is, 'If we've successfully got to our fifties or sixties without cardiovascular disease, then the focus should be on strength training to maintain our quality of life for as long as possible – to get off the toilet, out of bed, to be able to walk up and down the stairs ourselves for as long as possible independently. Weight training is not just about pumping muscle, or going to the gym, bulking up and lifting weights. The simple squat snacks and sit and stands are mimicking being able to get off the toilet unaided and save the embarrassment we feel once we are unable to help ourselves.' It's exactly what I say in my free Feel Good workouts. Ageing is inevitable, but it's about maintaining the best quality of life we can for as long as possible – and a lot of it is within our control. See more about strength training on page 61.

Find something you enjoy

Professor Murphy and I were in full agreement that we wish people could bottle up the feeling after movement or exercise and use that for the times when you're not feeling like moving and are lacking motivation. Whatever you do, it has to be something you enjoy for you to regularly do it. That's why I have provided so many snacks in this book for you to choose from, as we all have different taste buds. For example, HIIT is often daunting for many people. It may be best to add it in after you've got used to a certain level of exercise (and I give lots of low-impact and quick options to get you started). My message is that we mustn't neglect strength training, and that's why I go into it in the most detail, as I really want you to focus on it when selecting your snacks.

Sit less, move more

One of the biggest issues we face nowadays is the impact of sedentary lifestyles, with sitting being the silent killer, summed up by the phrase 'sitting is the new smoking'. Exercise snacking encourages regular movement throughout the day. This is less likely to result in long amounts of time sitting, which are linked to slow metabolism, high blood pressure, poor blood sugar control and a decrease in the body's ability to effectively break down fat. Sedentary lifestyles are also linked with disease and early death.

Any sort of movement that breaks up prolonged periods of sitting is beneficial – just do what you can, when you can. A study in 2020 found that people who sat for about 8 to 10 hours daily, but managed to do about 11 minutes of moderate-to-vigorous exercise a day, were less likely to die prematurely than those who only got about 2 minutes of exercise a day.

Sitting all day can put you at risk of health issues, even if you exercise daily. I think this is really important to note: it's not that great for you to do an hour's workout in the morning and then spend the rest of the day sitting. Prolonged sitting almost cancels out any health benefits from a daily workout. In fact, a study published by the Mayo Clinic found that 2 hours of sitting could cancel out the benefits of 20 minutes of exercise. People who exercise but spend the rest of their day sitting, still had elevated levels of blood sugar, cholesterol and body fat.

Do you work out for 30–60 minutes in the morning? But then spend the rest of the day staring at your computer, followed by settling in front of the television at night? If you answered yes to both questions, then you meet the definition of what scientists call 'an active couch potato'. This is common, don't worry, but it's something I want to raise awareness of – and change. The lesson from this research is that the goal is to be sitting less; we need to move lightly and often. Try to move more, however you can, whenever you can, and in ways you enjoy.

By taking activity snack breaks, little and often, we can break up sitting time and improve our health. That's where the power and importance of exercise snacking comes in. So keep moving and snacking through the day!

Backed by science

All the science, research and studies referenced in this book can be found in the notes on my website https://feelgoodwithlavina.com/thefeelgoodfix.

- The benefits of exercise snacking were first outlined in a 2014 study. It found that 'dosing exercise as brief, intense exercise snacks before a main meal is a time-efficient and effective approach to improve glycaemic control for individuals with insulin resistance'.
- Other studies show that exercise snacks/small bursts can lead to a 40 per cent reduction in blood sugar and blood fat levels.
- A 2019 study found that workouts lasting under 15 minutes, which included a warm-up, cool-down, and less than 5 minutes of vigorous exercise, could improve blood sugar control as well as heart and lung function (which help reduce the risks of type 2 diabetes and cardiovascular disease).
- Another 2019 study found that inactive adults who completed just 3 bursts of sprint cycling lasting 20 seconds had the same improvements to their cardiovascular fitness as those who completed the workout in 10 minutes, which suggests that spreading your training throughout the day is just as good for your heart.
- A small study in 2021 suggested that working out in snappy 4 second bursts for less than 15 minutes a day could boost your cardio fitness and provide benefits that

are equal to a longer workout, and may offset the risks of a sedentary lifestyle.

- A study published in January 2022 found that performing short bursts (1 minute or less) of vigorous exercise – which they referred to as 'exercise snacks' – at intervals throughout the day was a 'feasible, well-tolerated and time-efficient approach' to improving heart and lung health and reducing the impact of a sedentary lifestyle on cardiometabolic health.
- A study from December 2022 found that just 1 minute bursts of intense activity performed 3 or 4 times a day can boost overall health to reduce the risk of premature death by up to 49 per cent.

One of the biggest research projects is currently being undertaken by Loughborough University over six years. The team has devised a programme called Snacktivity™, aimed at getting the sedentary population moving more. The goal is still to hit the NHS-backed guidelines of 30 minutes of moving a day, but rather than setting aside a formal half-hour on an exercise mat, you accumulate moving minutes over the day.

Just like my method, rather than seeing exercise as a daunting block of time, Snacktivity™ adopts a 'whole day' approach. Given the lack of success in encouraging inactive populations to achieve larger bursts of physical activity as stated in the government guidelines, it's great to see that research like this is being funded. The team say in their published papers that recent UK and WHO guidance has discussed the merits of short bursts of physical activity. However, guidance that sets large behavioural goals for physical activity has not been successful in supporting the public to become sufficiently physically active, and a 'one size fits all' approach to physical activity guidelines may not be optimal.

I spoke to their lead, Professor Amanda Daley, about how they envisage it being implemented. The Snacktivity™ intervention is designed to be delivered by health care professionals and will take five minutes to deliver within the usual NHS consultations. The Snacktivity™ programme (funded by a grant from the National Institute for Health and Care Research) is also going to investigate if this approach is particularly appropriate for specific populations such as the elderly, pregnant women, and people with chronic diseases, who may be reluctant to engage in physical activity. Over the next few years, they will explore all these ideas and conduct research on whether this approach is acceptable, effective, or easier to sustain over time. 'Behaviour change and habit formation are best achieved through the gradual building of task self-efficacy, celebrating small successes,' say the Loughborough researchers.

11 minutes to change your life

One of the most exciting pieces of research for me is a 2022 study published in the *British Journal of Sports Medicine*, which states that just 11 minutes of daily exercise can substantially reduce a person's risk of early death, and help prevent heart disease, stroke and some cancers. Researchers found that 1 in 10 premature deaths could be prevented if people exercised for 75 minutes per week, or 11 minutes per day.

Although results were even better for those who exercised for 150 minutes weekly, or 30 minutes daily, 5 times a week (the recommended guidelines for physical activity to date); nearly 16 per cent of all premature deaths could be avoided if sedentary people achieved this metric, the review says. But this is hard to achieve in our modern lifestyles.

These new findings of doing just 11 minutes a day are great news, as most people find the idea of 150 minutes of moderate-intensity physical activity a week a bit daunting. People who did just 75 minutes of moderate to vigorous exercise each week (i.e. 11 minutes a day) were 17 per cent less likely to develop cardiovascular disease and 7 per cent less likely to develop cancer, as compared to those who were sedentary. (Those who exercised for 150 minutes per week saw a 27 per cent lower risk of cardiovascular disease and a 12 per cent lower risk of cancer. It's worth pointing out that these benefits started to plateau, however, as the amount of weekly physical activity continued to increase. Any benefit in exercising for more than 300 minutes weekly was uncertain, researchers said.)

Up until now, I have always encouraged everyone to start off small and gradually build up to hitting the UK government guidelines for physical activity, aiming to do at least 150 minutes of moderate-intensity activity a week or 75 minutes of vigorous-intensity activity a week (or a combination of both), plus a minimum of two strength training workouts a week. Hitting these guidelines for physical activity can reduce your risk of developing many long-term chronic conditions (such as heart disease, stroke, type 2 diabetes and cancer) by up to 50 per cent, reduce the risk of osteoarthritis by up to 83 per cent, and lower your risk of dementia, depression and even early death by up to 30 per cent.

The studies confirm that short bursts of activity do count, and they back up what I've been saying about exercise snacking. I really want to reframe the way we look at fitness, as aiming for 11 minutes is much more achievable and realistic. The studies not only confirm that there are immediate benefits from short bouts of exercise, but also that exercise snacking helps to combat chronic conditions, and promotes long-term adaptations and fitness changes. Exercise helps lower inflammation in the body, decreases fat tissue, and helps with hormone regulation and sleep – all of these things in tandem will keep you healthier overall. Exercise boosts your mental fitness too, from your self-esteem to your mood and energy, as well as reducing your risk of stress, depression and chronic illnesses like dementia and Alzheimer's disease.

It's great news that you don't have to exercise for longer to reap more benefits, especially when we are all battling to find time. 11 minutes a day is the perfect starting goal. If you want to hit 30 minutes a day then, of course, go for it! But be reassured in knowing that 11 minutes is of great benefit, and that's a great target to aim for.

Exercise snacking is the healthiest type of snacking around

How to start

Identify and define your 'why'

This is something I have asked every client I have ever trained. It's important to think about your 'why' – the deep-seated reason you want to do this – as this will help your mindset and motivation. You can't always rely on external or short-term factors, such as holidays, to motivate you, especially as you age. These come and go, we are all getting older, and our bodies are changing and facing challenges. Midlife gives us an opportunity to gain control of our health and think more long term. Defining your why will give you a personal or emotional investment in your goals.

Some soul searching is required. I want you to think about and write down your why. Go deep! Once you have worked out your why, then the who, what, when, where and how become so much easier to figure out. There's no right or wrong, this is just an invitation to reflect on your why.

I periodically ask myself this same question, as it has changed over time. I have many reasons why I choose to put health first. I work out because I actually *love* it, and enjoy it! I love being strong and I like to see how far I can push myself, so I set personal goals. I exercise to stay fit and healthy, both physically and mentally. For my bones, brain, heart, mental and long-term health. It helps me cope with day-to-day challenges and alleviates my worries. When I train, it gives me my me-time to refuel, refocus and clear my mind. It actually makes me *feel good* and then I am in a better mood and energized for my four boys. It helps me manage my perimenopausal symptoms and gives me self-worth, confidence and empowerment. Over the last few years, my why has changed from being focused on how I look, to how I feel mentally and the importance of exercise to my long-term health.

Your why may be to enjoy running around with your kids or grandkids. It may be to manage your menopausal weight gain. It may be to look good and feel good. It may be to help with the symptoms of the menopause, like alleviating anxiety, stress, joint pain, or to sleep better. It may be to help prevent osteoporosis, dementia or type 2 diabetes, which may be in your family. Or it may be something very personal.

Once you have it, write it out! Post it somewhere you'll see it every day, for your reminder. That way, when times get tough, you will remember why you started, your reasons for setting out in the first place, and why you shouldn't quit.

Start off small

It's imperative to remember that when you're starting out on a feel-good journey of your own, you take small steps at first towards your strength training, exercise and healthy lifestyle. Consider your personal goals and limitations. Don't worry about anyone else; this is the time to focus on you.

This book, and my approach to your midlife and beyond, is about reclaiming your health, understanding your menopause symptoms, and tuning in to your hormones. I will give you tools to navigate the journey and work out what you need and enjoy.

The ancient Chinese philosopher Lao-tzu stated, 'A journey of a thousand miles begins with a single step.' This mindset can be applied to practically any of your sought-after goals, including exercise and lifestyle. This particular journey can seem extremely daunting, so start with one simple Feel Good snack. It's about using your Feel Good toolkit to empower and educate yourself so you understand how to take control of your health, start off with small changes and create habits that will last.

Snack-size SMART goal setting

A step at a time also applies to goal setting, which is a great way to keep on track and stay motivated. Look at the bigger picture – if you know where you want to get to, you can work out how you are going to get there. You can then set more specific medium- and short-term 'SMART' goals to help you achieve your long-term goals.

Make every goal a SMART goal: Specific, Measurable, Attainable, Relevant and Timely. I actually learnt about, and used, SMART goal setting in my previous career as a project manager. I love applying it now to wellness and all aspects of my life.

I want us to reframe the way we think of goals and exercise. Don't make it all or nothing. Rather than setting unrealistic long-term goals, my advice is to set small, achievable goals to help you stay on track, not too big that you set yourself up for failure. You can build up from there and celebrate successes along the way.

Trust me, I know that being a woman, going through life phases such as perimenopause and menopause isn't always easy. But we can approach these stages positively and get through it!

You won't reach your goal overnight. Find one small step you can take today towards achieving your goal. Small steps equal big, lasting results, but only if you start taking them 'one step at a time'.

Consistency, perseverance and patience for long-term lifestyle changes

I am a big promoter of the mentality that wellness is a journey, not a quick transformation. I want it to be sustainable and become part of your long-term lifestyle. I've been through it, so I know there will be ups and downs – it's about consistency, patience and perseverance. Trust me, those feel-good endorphins (the happy hormones we release every time we exercise) will really help boost your mood to help you enjoy the journey.

Remember to celebrate your wins. Rather than focusing on just the physical results, notice and celebrate the non-physical positive changes derived from exercising. For example, the improvements in your mood, stress levels, mental health, energy, strength, sleep, fitness, stamina, flexibility, relationships, work, family and life-style. Plus the health metrics (blood pressure, resting heart rate, cholesterol levels, etc.) and the health benefits of reducing the risk of so many common chronic illnesses (including ones we can't always see).

Don't compare your journey with anyone else's. We are all individual and different, and we face so many challenges with hormones, perimenopause and menopause, so always be kind to yourself. By investing in your physical and mental health, you can celebrate what our amazing bodies do for us.

Motivation hacks

How do I stay motivated? It's a question I always get asked. I hope these easy, fun concepts help with your motivation to exercise.

- Schedule your snacks: add them to your diary like you would an appointment.
- Set a reminder/alarm (so you don't forget if you have peri/menopausal brain fog).
- Start off small: keep it varied.
- Dress for the part, if wearing your workout gear makes it more likely to make it happen. But you don't actually need to be in workout clothes for my snacks!
- Keep your mat, trainers, tins/bottles/dumbbells, resistance band visible and ready in places where you can use them.
- Make it social: you could exercise with a friend, family or work colleague, or have a snacking buddy, which can really help with accountability.
- Share your snacks on social media (and tag me!) to keep you accountable and motivate friends to join you.
- Do it for someone else: you could pick a cause or join a challenge so you have a long-term goal, and doing it for charity is so rewarding. Keep a diary, record your progress and how it makes you feel, focus on the overall health benefits of exercise.
- Celebrate your wins and reward yourself. See the menu of self-care nibbles on page 269.

How to use this book

I want this book to be your buddy, your companion, a handy guide that gives you a practical and relatable Feel Good plan and a pick 'n' mix menu of exercise and lifestyle snacks, where you select what you fancy and what you can fit into your busy life, in order to treat your body and mind. *You* are in control. Just aim to pick 'n' mix snacks to hit your 11 minutes a day.

The book is divided into snacks for physical health, mental health, and for life. You can flick through the book and stop to read about one of my snacks in detail or choose a specific practice or workout, which you can then start and do anywhere. There are mood menus at the back of the book (on page 365), where you can select whatever you fancy. Satisfy your cravings and binge on these. You can even combine a few snack recipes and make a meal of it. Depending on your energy, body and time available, you can select one that matches how you feel using the icons on each snack.

I want to make snacking as easy and appealing as possible, so I have filmed many of the more complex snacks for you to follow along. All you have to do is use your smart phone or tablet and scan the QR code on the page. This will take you to my YouTube channel where you can simply hit the play button!

Your phone or tablet's built-in camera app can scan QR codes, and it's as easy as taking a photo.

- Open the camera app and hold your phone, so the QR code appears in the viewfinder.

- Your phone should recognize the QR code and give you a notification.
- Tap the notification to open the link associated with the QR code, taking you straight to my YouTube channel.

Don't worry, I have also added in short descriptions of all the exercises as little reminders of how to do them, just in case you don't want to scan the QR code for whatever reason.

As you get used to snacking, you can build up to following your own 7-day snacking plan. Just like a weekly meal plan, I'd love you to have a weekly Feel Good Plan pinned on your fridge.

There is no right or wrong, and ideally you will hit the 11 minutes of exercise a day and then everything on top is a bonus! But remember, even if you hit less than 11 minutes it's still effective and counts, so be kind to yourself. *Everything* counts!

Selecting your snacks

The snacks are ordered by time so you can choose accordingly, based on whether you have 1/3/5/10 minutes – and of course you can combine them to hit 11 minutes a day. Look out for the symbols on each page that will tell you what type of exercise this is and what it's good for.

Length of exercise:

🕐 1min   1 minute
🕐 3min   3 minutes
🕐 5min   5 minutes
🕐 10min 10 minutes

Focus of exercise:

Mobility
Cardio
Strength
Stretch
Balance
Brain
Journal

Breath
Nature
Sleep
Recovery
Social
Work

Each snack is like a recipe for success, with a full method, benefits, next steps (suggestions to stack your snacks, and opportunities to 'piggyback' on to existing behaviours and habits, so you're prompted) and top tips.

Really, there are no strict rules. This approach to exercise, lifestyle and mindfulness is all about doing what you can, when you can, in the life that you lead. However you use this book, I hope you have fun, and come to understand that feeling good is closer and easier than you think. Let's find and embrace the joy in midlife and beyond!

Sample snack plans

Here are some examples of how you can put together your own weekly plan together using the snacks in this book. The idea is to select different snacks from each of the areas in this book, to get a variety, try them out and see what you enjoy. Just be sure not to work the same muscle groups too much, so they have time to rest, grow and recover.

You can do different snacks every day. Or you may love some snacks as a morning/evening/daily ritual that you want to keep on repeat. There are no rules, it's completely flexible, and your snack plan can be tailor made to suit your schedule and mood, but it's always helpful to have a plan to aim for.

Pick 'n' mix: pick your own snacks to treat your body and mind from the mood menus on page 365.

11 minute sample plans

Example 1

Cold Water Snack   1 min
10 Second Balance Snack   1 min
Wake-Up Stretch Snack   3 mins
Feel Good Walk Snack   3 mins

Full Body Strength Snack   1 min
Mindful Minute 5.5 Breath
   Snack   1 min
Happy Jar Snack   1 min

Example 2

Fitness Salutation Snack   3 mins
Full Body Strength Snack   5 mins
Dose of Vitamin G Snack   1 min

Stair Snack   1 min
Best Back Stretch Snack   1 min

Example 3

Daily Affirmation Snack   1 min
Mindful Minute 4-6 Breath
   Snack   1 min
Feel Good Hug Snack   1 min
10 Second Balance Snack   1 min
Stair Snack   1 min

Cold Water Snack   1 min
Shoulder Floss Snack   1 min
Full Body Strength Snack   1 min
HIIT Snack   1 min
Pelvic Floor Snack   1 min
Best Back Stretch Snack   1 min

Example 4: exercise snacks only

Shoulder Floss Snack   1 min
10 Second Balance Snack   1 min
Pelvic Floor Snack   1 min
Stair Snack   1 min

HIIT Snack   1 min
Full Body Strength Snack
   (pick 1 exercise)   5 mins
Feel Good Finish Snack   1 min

Example 5: upper body exercise snacks

Upper Body Mobility
Snack   5 mins
Upper Body Strength
Snack   5 mins

Best Back Stretch
Snack   1 min

Example 6: lower body exercise snacks

Lower Body Mobility
Snack   5 mins
Lower Body Strength
Snack   5 mins

End of Day Stretch Snack
(pick 1 exercise)   1 min

Example 7: at work snacks

Desk Reset Snack   1 min
Stand Snack   1 min
Seated Strength Snack   5 mins
Tech Neck Stretch Snack   1 min

Stair Snack   1 min
HIIT Snack   1 min
Best Back Stretch Snack   1 min

30 minute sample plans

Example 1

Wake-Up Stretch Snack   3 min
10 Second Balance Snack   1 min
Mindful Minute 4-6 Breath
Snack   1 min
3 Goals for the Day Snack
3 mins

Sunshine and Grounding
Snacks, combined with
either Superbrain Snack or
Feel Good Walk Snack
10 mins
Cold Water Snack   1 min

Full Body Strength Snack   5 mins

Stair Snack   1 min

HIIT Snack   3 mins

End of Day Stretch Snack (pick
  one move)   1 min

Pelvic Floor Snack   1 min

Example 2

3 Goals for the Day Snack
  3 mins

Pelvic Floor Snack   1 min

Fitness Salutation Snack   3 mins

Upper Body Mobility
  Snack   5 mins

Upper Body Strength
  Snack   10 mins

Core Snack   5 mins

Shoulder Floss Snack   1 min

Feel Good Finish Snack   1 min

Feel Good Hug Snack   1 min

60 minute sample plans

Example 1

Wake-Up Stretch Snack   3 mins

Yoga Balance Snack   3 mins

Alternate Nostril Breathing
  Snack   3 mins

3 Goals for the Day Snack
  3 mins

Feel Good Walk Snack   10 mins

Cold Water Snack   1 min

Stair Snack   1 min

HIIT Snack   5 mins

Mobility snack (select a few
  from upper and lower body
  mobility snacks) or Fitness
  Salutation Snack   5 mins

Upper Body Strength Snack
  5 mins

Lower Body Strength Snack
  5 mins

Core Snack   5 mins

Write Away Your Worries Snack
  5 mins

Pelvic Floor Snack and 10 Second
  Balance Snack combo   1 min

End of Day Stretch Snack
  5 mins

Example 2

Train the Brain Snack   10 mins

Sunshine Snack   10 mins

Full Body Mobility Snack
   10 mins

Lower Body Strength and Cardio
   Snack   10 mins

Full Body Stretch Snack
   (combine Post-Workout
   Upper and Lower Body
   Stretch Snacks)   10 mins

Heat Snack   10 mins

Remember, it's *your* Feel Good journey. There is no right or wrong. Listen to your body, and be kind to yourself.

You could write up your ideal plan for the upcoming week on a Sunday night, or you could complete this as you go through the week. Don't beat yourself up if it doesn't go to 'plan'. Just take each day as it comes and stay in tune with your peri/menopause symptoms. Every little bit counts!

Feel Good Physically

Feel Good Fitness Prescription

The Feel Good Fitness Prescription provides a holistic, balanced approach for optimum health, longevity and long-term sustainable results. It combines mobility, cardio, strength training, stretching and balance snacks. These are the foundations of my Feel Good approach, and I will explain each of these in detail.

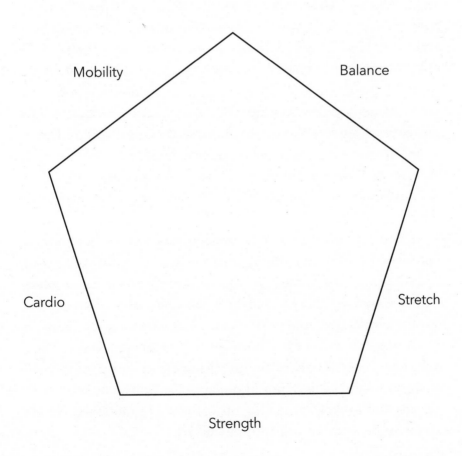

Mobility

Joint aches and pains can be one of the biggest challenges to starting exercise, especially as we go through the menopause. Mobility helps our joints move actively through their full range of motion and is critical for healthy movement. I like to use mobility in a few different ways – as a warm-up exercise, but equally to snack on it throughout the day, especially to break up long periods of sitting and to ease away any tightness, aches and pains. Looking after your joints is so underrated, but once you make it part of your daily routine, like stretching, I think you'll not only love it but reap the benefits too. Motion really is lotion!

The benefits of mobility training include increased performance, strength and power, faster recovery, injury reduction and prevention, better posture and general well-being. Like stretching, mobility takes time and regular practice; by slowly incorporating mobility snacks you will hopefully begin to alleviate any pain or discomfort in your joints and they will get stronger, become more supple and looser.

If you get into the habit of moving your joints through their full range of motion without added weight (i.e. just using your bodyweight), you'll improve your ability to move those joints during weighted and high-impact exercises, as well as day-to-day functional movements. Functional movements are the main seven movement patterns that your body relies on to get things done every day, not just when exercising: squat, lunge, push, pull, hinge, twist and walk. Think about how you pull a box off a shelf, squat down to pick something up, carry your grandchildren, get up from the floor, or walk around all day.

Regular mobility training provides benefits in ways that a quick warm-up cannot. During mobility training, blood is being moved to the surrounding tissues. Synovial fluid, the fluid in our joints that helps them to glide freely, is carried into the working joints. This synovial fluid loosens and lubricates the joints (isn't that amazing?).

By including simple but effective mobility snacks frequently in your Feel Good toolkit, I guarantee your performance in your exercises will improve. It will reduce existing or potential chances of injury, and you will feel so good for it. They're ideal to do anytime of the day. I see mobility as a form of self-care too, and the moves will help open and de-stress your body and your mind.

Explore the menus of snacks on page 366, or look for the mobility icon in the snack sections to treat your joints. There are even some gentle seated options for those who are less mobile or anyone who is chained to their desk. Get snacking and get mobilizing! If you need one to start with, try the Fitness Salutation Snack on page 124, I swear by this one.

Cardio

Aerobic activity and cardiovascular training play such an important role for women during peri/menopause, especially with the greater risk of heart disease (see page 20).

The current UK government guidelines for physical activity are to aim for 150 minutes of moderate-intensity cardiovascular activity or 75 minutes of vigorous-intensity cardiovascular activity, or a combination of both, per week.

But now we know that even 11 minutes of (moderate-intensity) movement a day has amazing benefits for your long-term health. So I'd encourage you to aim for this – and then, by all means, build up.

Cardio activity, comes in so many forms. The most important thing is to do something that you enjoy.

- *Examples of moderate-intensity cardio*: walking, light jogging, cycling, swimming, dancing or gardening
  The aim is to raise your heart rate to the point where your breathing increases, you feel warmer and can maintain a conversation but can't sing a song.
- *Examples of vigorous-intensity cardio*: running, HIIT training, sprint, boxing or stair snacking (see page 106)
  You should feel like you are working hard, short/out of breath, your heart rate should be high and beating faster. You may struggle to maintain a conversation easily, let alone sing a song.

Strength training

If there's one form of exercise I want you to start after reading this book, or to focus on even more, it's to snack regularly on strength training.

Whatever age we are, it is crucial for our health that we lift weights, plus it is a powerful tool to kick those peri/menopause symptoms (as I have found) and essential to optimize women's long-term health.

Strength training can be defined as any physiological movement that uses bodyweight or equipment to engage your muscles. It works by putting stress and load on the bones and muscles, and as a result, they respond positively by getting stronger.

Strength training is important, to maintain and strengthen muscles, bones and joints, to build lean muscle (to reduce the risk of osteoporosis), as well as to improve balance and keep heart and brain fit. Regular strength training can also help you reduce body fat (the common 'menopot'), maintain a healthy weight and burn calories more efficiently. Strength training is often the missing piece in the wellness jigsaw. In my opinion, it trumps cardio since the more muscle mass we have, the more calories we burn, even at rest. With effective weight management we also reduce the risk of so many other chronic midlife illnesses, such as heart disease, dementia, type 2 diabetes (the more muscle you have, the better your insulin sensitivity, even at rest).

What's more, in addition to potentially lowering your weight, resistance workouts include functional moves emphasizing power and balance, which enhance strength and stability, reduce pain and the risk of potential falls. This helps us maintain our independence as we age and enhances our quality of life by improving our ability to do everyday activities.

It is beneficial to start strength training as early as possible, although it's never too late to start. You begin to lose muscle mass (sarcopenia) after the age of thirty, and you can lose as much as 3 per cent to 5 per cent of muscle mass each decade approximately (but even up to 1 per cent to 3 per cent of muscle mass every year), unless you engage in regular resistance training. Furthermore, during perimenopause itself, the loss of muscle and bone density accelerates. When you hit the menopause, the rate at which you lose muscle mass increases substantially. In a 2021 study, researchers found that compared to women in early perimenopause, those in late perimenopause had 10 per cent less muscle mass in their arms and legs. Once you go into post-menopause, the oestrogen loss accelerates and the decrease in muscle and bone mass is turbo-charged.

Strength training also has a positive and protective effect against heart disease, which we are more susceptible to in menopause. One study shows that menopausal women who strength trained regularly had fewer inflammatory chemicals linked with heart disease. And there's also evidence to suggest that resistance training reduces the risk of someone having a heart attack or stroke. Strength training and exercise also helps improve our immunity as it releases immune-boosting proteins called cytokines.

So the message I want to shout loud and clear is that, as women, we must all be doing strength training regularly, whatever our age. As my Feel Good method is about making it accessible to everyone, of all ages and abilities, this book includes seated strength snacks also, and bodyweight training is always a great way to start.

Progressive overload

The aim with strength training is to make the exercise progressively harder, gradually over time, as your strength increases and your body adapts, while maintaining perfect form. To strengthen your muscles, you need to move them against some resistance. Increasing muscle resistance can be done by adding a load/weight for the muscles to work against.

With weights remember not to go heavy too quickly; perfect your form, feel each move, and progress gradually over time. Start with just your bodyweight, then add light weights (dumbbells/tins/plastic bottles/weighted rucksack/safe household objects) and increase weights over time.

You can also progressively overload by increasing reps and sets, varying the tempo, making the exercise harder, reducing rest periods, and even going slower on the way down.

The magic of myokines

When you contract your muscles, it secretes these magical chemicals called myokines, which are thought to have positive effects on everything from cognitive function to blood sugar, to killing cancer cells, to boosting your metabolism and mental health, as well as being anti-inflammatory! The name 'myokines' actually means 'set into motion by your muscles'. When you exercise, your body naturally pushes myokines out of your muscles. Then, they enter the bloodstream and cross over the blood–brain barrier, acting as antidepressants.

Therefore, when people exercise, they feel better. Scientists have dubbed them 'hope molecules' as they alleviate anxiety and change the structure of your brain to make you more resilient to stress and trauma.

I really wanted to share this science with you, as many women struggle to find the motivation to move their body, or are experiencing persistent sadness, anxiety or low mood. I have faith that these hope molecules can give you hope and help make a positive change for you. It's not just about using exercise to make yourself feel better when you're down, but using it so you don't feel so low in the first place.

Ladies, get lifting!

As mentioned earlier, we need to aim to hit the physical activity guidelines of 150 mins of moderate or 75 minutes of vigorous aerobic activity a week (through our cardio snacks). But in addition, the guidelines around the world advise us to strength train at least 2 or 3 times a week. I personally recommend snacking on strength training up to 5 days of the week (targeting different body parts). It doesn't have to be a long strength training session each time, and you definitely don't need fancy equipment or gym membership. You just need to start off small, with your bodyweight, then build up progressively, light and slow (constantly challenging yourself as you get stronger over time), and keep it consistent. I'll show you how with the strength snacks in this book.

Lifting weights can help by promoting muscle growth and strength, yet only a fraction of people over the age of seventy-five perform strength training at least twice a week. But researchers and experts say you're never too old to start, even if you have arthritis, heart disease, dementia or osteoporosis.

Lifting weights for less than an hour a week may reduce your risk of a heart attack or stroke by between 40 and 70 per cent, according to a study by Iowa State University. This research states that you don't have to invest a lot of time in lifting weights to lower your risk of cardiovascular disease – less than 5 minutes could be effective, which is so encouraging.

Take your pick from the exercise snacks with the strength icon to indulge in some strength snacks.

Strength training glossary

I've tried to keep the terminology in this book as simple as possible but here are some common terms you might not be familiar with.

Bodyweight

This means just you, not using any additional weights.

Reps

A repetition is one complete motion of an exercise – like the movement down and up in the squat or biceps curl. I'd recommend aiming for 8–12 reps (to build and grow muscle – hypertrophy), but do as many/little as you can while maintaining perfect form.

Sets

A group of consecutive repetitions (for example, 8–10 reps in a set).

Tempo

The rate or pace at which a rep is performed. The slower the tempo, the more time under tension for the muscles, so it's a great way to progress and get stronger too. (Especially on the eccentric (lowering and lengthening) part of the move – think of weight lowering, not just weight lifting.)

Super sets

Where you do two exercises back to back, without taking a rest in between.

EMOM

Each Move On the Minute – a fun way to snack by doing a few different exercises/snacks with a timer and seeing how much you can do in a minute. (Use the time left over before the end of each minute to rest in between.)

Don't focus on your weight on the scales, focus on the weight you're lifting

Bone health and osteoporosis

Osteoporosis is when bones become thinner and less dense, causing them to fracture more easily. Menopause significantly speeds up bone loss and increases the risk of osteoporosis. Research indicates that up to 20 per cent of bone loss can happen during these stages. One in two post-menopausal women will have osteoporosis, and most will suffer a fracture during their lifetime.

Strength training targets the bones of the hips, the spine and the wrists – which are most likely to fracture. Here are some alarming statistics: it is reported that, worldwide, 9 million women annually experience a fracture, resulting in an osteoporosis fracture every three seconds. Nearly 75 per cent of all hip fractures occur in women. Osteoporosis takes a huge personal and economic toll. Did you know that the number of women who go on to die from fractures is similar to the number of women who die from breast cancer? Hip fractures cause the most morbidity, with an increase in reported mortality rates: between 20 and 24 per cent of patients will die within a year of fracturing their hip, and 50 per cent will no longer be able to live independently for the rest of their lives. So it's huge in terms of personal impact, but it's also a huge burden on the healthcare system. The NHS spends £4.4 billion a year treating and managing the effects of osteoporosis.

Muscle loss and bone loss go hand in hand, especially during the menopause transition, when both tend to accelerate. Building and preserving muscle mass is also key to reducing the risks of osteoporosis, which is vital at this stage in our lives and as we age. Osteoporosis is preventable (which is why I want women to start young, by their thirties) but strength training specifically has been shown to help prevent bone loss and maintain bone mass, even in those who already have osteoporosis. Weight bearing and muscle strengthening exercises apply stress to the bones, which in turn respond by renewing themselves to make them stronger too.

When your muscles pull on your bones, it gives your bones work to do. Your bones respond by renewing themselves and maintaining or improving their strength.

One study shows that women who exercise regularly can reduce their risk of getting osteoporosis after the menopause. And another study which looked at women who already had post-menopausal osteoporosis found that women who strength trained twice a week had better bone density than those who did not. Therefore, it is key to do strength training exercises at least 2 or 3 times a week, but I encourage you to do my strength snacks as often as you can, alternating muscle groups so you're not training the same ones on consecutive days. As your muscles get stronger, they pull harder, meaning your bones are more likely to become stronger. Research studies have shown that progressive strength training (see 'Progressive overload' on page 63) is likely to be the best type of muscle strengthening exercise for increasing bone strength.

Stretching

Stretching is vital but often skipped! When we lift weights we actually create tiny tears in the muscles, and stretching after your session helps to circulate fresh blood and feed the muscles with the nutrients needed for repair and recovery. Its role is essential in preventing injuries, boosting performance, and often healing existing injuries too. Stretching increases flexibility and helps keep us mobile. Look at how super mobile babies and young children are, but we lose this as we grow into adults. When we stop stretching, we lose capacity in movement, which means we are able to move less; we are functionally less able to do everyday stuff like pick up a sock from the floor, scratch our back, or even climb stairs efficiently.

It's also super important to stretch out our sedentary lifestyles. The more we sit, the more our muscles are shortening, which in turn causes more tightness, pain, poor posture and restriction of movement. Most of us think stretching is only for athletes or gymnasts. But the fact is, it is essential for all of us.

Stretching makes us feel good

Stretching is not just about keeping the muscles strong or improving our flexibility. It also has the power to improve our mental health. Stretching increases blood flow to the brain and throughout the body. When we stretch, our body releases the magical feel-good hormones called endorphins – yes, as per my branding and the title of this book! Endorphins are responsible for triggering the brain receptors that increase positive feelings and reduce pain.

In addition to helping you feel relaxed, stretching increases your body's levels of serotonin, which is the hormone that can help stabilize your mood and reduce stress. A study found that implementing stretching exercises at work also reduced anxiety and exhaustion while increasing vitality and mental health. See more tips in the work chapter on page 331.

Stretching lengthens and elongates the muscles to aid recovery and can reduce the delayed onset muscle soreness (DOMS) you may feel after a workout. From increasing our blood circulation and boosting our mood, to improving the quality of sleep, stretching can also do wonders for our mental well-being. Stretching has been proven to be one of the simplest and most effective ways to reduce stress and calm the mind in order to find emotional and mental balance. So when we go through anxiety, stress and fatigue from workload, menopause or juggling the demands of life, a little self-care by stretching can do us a world of good.

Please consider adding stretching to your daily arsenal of tools to battle those long, hard days of being a woman. It's an integral part of the menopause Feel Good toolkit.

Stretching can boost your strength and muscle mass

Research published in the *Journal of Applied Physiology* revealed that stretching has much the same effect on muscles as weight training does. Both stretching and lifting cause micro tears in the muscle tissue, which stimulate your muscle cells to produce growth factors. These growth factors promote the manufacture of new muscle fibres, and can boost your weight-lifting potential.

Start stretching

Scatter stretches throughout the day, to treat yourself and alleviate the demands of our modern-day lifestyle and time spent sitting. Remember, there's no limit! One of the best things about stretching is that it takes very little time and can be done anywhere.

Stretching for a few minutes is such a good place to start. If you are tight, use your breath to help relieve any areas of tension – deep breathing really helps you through your stretches. Make it into a habit and hopefully it will become a tool that you love, like I do now.

There are so many short stretches in this book, but it's helpful to stretch regularly to leverage its full potential. Select some stretch snacks and piggyback on to your daily activities. You can stack the stretch snacks and even work your way up to a goal of, say, 10 minutes of daily stretching. I'm sure you'll gain noticeable results from it.

Balance

A key component of my Feel Good Fitness Prescription is balance, as many people forget the importance of working on it. Studies have shown poor balance can be associated with serious health problems – as well as increased risks of falls as we get older. (See the section on osteoporosis on page 68 for more information on fractures.) With balance beginning to diminish from midlife onwards, from the age of forty-five, it is advisable to begin preventing the loss of balance sooner rather than later. It's like muscle: if you don't use it, you'll lose it. So unless you do something about it, your balance will deteriorate as you get older.

You should take a proactive approach to this as actively maintaining balance is likely to keep other health problems at bay. Start prevention in midlife and work on your balance before you need to, not after it becomes an issue. Once loss of balance begins, the problem can worsen quickly. Therefore, prevention is better than cure.

Balance exercises bring lots of advantages, from reducing your risk of falls (especially as you age) to correcting muscular imbalances, to strengthening your core muscles, helping to prevent injuries, giving better control over your body and posture, to increasing your performance in all other sports and exercises. Balance exercises improve body awareness and your proprioception (awareness of the position and movement of the body); they help with coordination, increase joint stability, correct muscular imbalances in the legs and improve reaction time.

Balance training is also good for the brain and it promotes neuromuscular coordination, which is the collaboration between your brain and your muscles. Balance training teaches the muscles to respond more quickly to messages from the brain and allows you to improve your fine motor skills and coordinating skills.

I think we take being able to balance for granted, until we actually start to lose our balance. You may notice how easy it used to be to stand on one leg and put a shoe on, but now you always need to sit down; or maybe that yoga tree pose used to be much simpler? Remember, we regularly need to stay in a one-legged posture, to get out of a car, to climb, or to descend a step or a stair. Although you may think balance issues arise much later on in life, many studies say balance starts to decline in your mid-forties, and it's not uncommon for menopausal women to experience disequilibrium, which is a feeling of unsteadiness and loss of balance, as if the room is spinning, even when you are still (which can be disorienting and very worrying at times). This can be due to fluctuating hormone levels that can affect blood pressure, circulation and the nervous system.

A lack of activity and sedentary lifestyles can cause a lack of balance. Sitting all day puts little strain on your balancing system and can make it hard for the brain to know what to do in situations that require you to be on your feet. Modern-day sedentary lifestyles, being less active and spending more time sitting behind screens and with tech, is causing our ability to balance to decline more rapidly than in previous generations. So it's essential we keep moving and get up regularly to snack on exercise!

Once balance begins to fail, the process can turn into a downward spiral as older people can't, or become afraid to, walk outside their homes. They can develop further imbalances as their muscles atrophy, which makes falls more likely.

A 2016 study found that older adults who did balance exercises for 6 weeks enhanced their balance control and gained confidence. The exercises also helped improve coordination, leg strength and ankle mobility.

There is a clear link between balance and longevity also. A 2016 study found that people's ability to sit on the floor and then stand up without using their hands or knees for support could predict their risk of death over the next six years. This is a simple exercise to try – give it a go!

Having good balance is a powerful predictor of how long and how healthily you will live. A 2022 study says that balancing on one leg for 10 seconds may predict the likelihood of living or dying. You're twice as likely to die in the next decade if you're unable to balance on one foot for 10 seconds. Conversely, the study suggests that your ability to balance on one foot points to longer life expectancy. (Head over to the 10 Second Balance Snack on page 86 for more details and extra challenges.)

I've been doing this balance snack every day while I brush my teeth (morning and night), it's become second nature and I can really see the improvement. The good news is that you can quickly improve your balance. And I'd encourage you to start sooner rather than later. Look for the balance icon and choose some snacks that take your fancy. Let's get working on that balance to keep active and confident, well into old age.

Desk Reset Snack

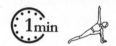

Sitting and slouching? Experiencing neck or back pain? This is the easiest trick to help you feel taller, more confident, and instantly improve your posture.

Research shows that we are more sedentary from midlife onwards, and our reliance on technology just exacerbates this. Physical inactivity in midlife, plus hunching over screens at our desks, is detrimental to our posture, our lower back, and can worsen the common menopausal joint pains.

Method

1. Visualize a desk shape.

2. Bring your shoulders up to your ears. Then take them backwards and down the spine (as if you've drawn a desk shape with your shoulders).

3. At the end, your shoulder blades should be set further down the spine, your chest should feel more open, and your back should be nice and straight, with your neck in a relaxed neutral position to your spine.

4. Repeat for a minute, or as long as you like!

Benefits

- Helps reverse rounding of the spine (kyphosis)
- Improves posture
- Relaxes any tension in your shoulders
- Reduces back pain and neck soreness
- Alleviates tech neck (the pain we get from looking down at devices)
- Lengthens the spine
- Makes you feel taller
- Boosts confidence and self-esteem.

Next steps

- If you have more time, stack this snack with a Feel Good Hug Snack on page 80 or a 1 minute Tech Neck Stretch Snack on page 78.

Tech Neck
Stretch Snack

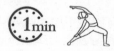

Is your neck sore from staring at your computer screen too long or bending down to look at your phone? Headaches, tight shoulders and upper back pain? Then try this quick 1 minute release.

Obviously, prevention is better than cure – so try to stop looking down at your devices. Instead, hold or set your phone at eye level (which is good for your arm muscles), and when you're at your computer, position your screen high enough so you can look straight at it, rather than down. Your spine should be in one straight line from the top of your head to your tail bone.

1. **Neck release**: Place your hand on the opposite ear, gently easing your other ear towards your shoulder (of the bent arm). You can place the other hand behind your back to deepen the stretch or tilt your head, maybe turning your nose towards the floor. Repeat on other side.

2. **Neck nods and nos**: Imagine you are saying a big yes by lifting your chin up and then bringing it down to your chest. Repeat a few times, easing out the front and nape of your neck. Also imagine you are saying no with your head by turning it left to right.

3. **Head circles**: Imagine you are drawing big circles with your chin, rotating your head in one direction a few times and then the other way.

Benefits

- Alleviates neck pain (always consult a physician if the pain is unbearable or persistent)
- Eases tension
- Improves posture

Next steps

- Stack on my feel-good Shoulder Floss Snack on page 84 or Desk/Sofa Snack on page 157.
- The TLC Back Snack on page 194 is a great one to help strengthen the important muscles in your back.

Top tips

- When doing the neck nods, I often imagine smiling and saying yes to positivity. And on the nos, saying no to negativity. A little mental hack to add to this snack.

Feel Good Hug Snack

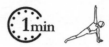

Feel good instantly by giving yourself a hug! Great for when you're feeling tight and you need a release – plus some self-love, which all of us women deserve!

A hug releases the 'love hormone' oxytocin, which is actually proven to make you feel good. Increased levels of oxytocin are attributed to happiness, but it also decreases levels of the stress hormone cortisol, which can improve the body's natural ability to fight illness, and give a boost to the immune system.

Method

1. Simply open your arms wide, arch your back, lift through your neck and chin, and tilt the base of your spine like you're sticking your bottom out.

2. Take a positive deep inhale here and then exhale as you wrap your arms round yourself/someone.

3. Focus on creating a C shape with your back, tuck the base of your spine in and under, opening out all the vertebrae in your back and bringing your chin to your chest.

4. Hug yourself and pat your back or give yourself a loving rub with your hands. Repeat as many times as you want.

Benefits

- Boosts mood
- Relieves stress
- Opens up the chest
- Relieves backaches
- Mobilizes the spine
- Releases the 'love hormone' oxytocin

Next steps

- Add in any Mindful Minute breath snack for more self-love and calm.
- Stack on with the Best Back Stretch Snack on page 104 for some back care.

Feel Good Finish Snack

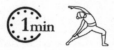

My famous Feel Good finish, a fabulous way to lengthen the body, unravel the spine, open out your body, breathe in positivity and release any tension.

When you link the simple lifting of the arms with your breath, it honestly captures positivity – and always brings a smile to my face – as well as being a great way to lengthen the spine and microdose your day with a feel-good move you can do anywhere (seated or standing).

Method

1. Stand or sit up straight and lengthen your arms down by your side.

2. Take a deep inhale, filled with positive thoughts, as you lift your straight arms, all the way up, with palms facing up so they meet above your head.

3. Breathe out any negativity, as you bring your arms back down to the starting position.

4. Repeat three times. On the final movement bring your hands down together in a prayer position to the centre of your chest, capturing all that positivity to your heart,

and then take a small bow. You could thank your body or even recite an affirmation or say *namaste*.

Benefits

- Calms your body and mind
- Increases feelings of positivity
- Releases stress or negative thoughts

Next steps

- Combine this with your Daily Affirmation Snack on page 277 for a great start to your day.
- Bolt this on to the end of your HIIT or strength snacks.

Top tips

- Lower the speed. If you take it nice and slow, your breaths will get deeper too and you'll probably feel more benefits.
- If you work at a desk or sofa, use this snack when you get up and go for a quick walk snack, to fill up your water bottle or get a cup of coffee. It's a great way to add this habit into your daily routine and it's not taking up more time in your already busy day.

Shoulder Floss Snack

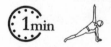

The 1 minute daily mobility drill I prescribe to help improve posture and loosen up tense shoulders, and keep your upper back and neck happy.

It's very common to not be able to do this with straight arms, so start by bending the arms and only go to the range of movement that works for you. Your arms don't need to go as low as your glutes behind you – build up to that over time. Ideally, your shoulder ball and socket joint will get full range of movement eventually to keep it nicely lubricated and functional.

Equipment

A long resistance band. If you don't have this, a pair of old tights, bathrobe tie or belt can work.

Method

1. Hold the band/pair of tights loosely between both hands, and raise your arms to the ceiling, while maintaining tension in the fabric. Now bring the band down over and behind your head, as far as you can go towards your bottom.

2. Then raise your hands and arms up, back over the front of your head, and bring them down in front of you again.

3. Keep flossing for up to 1 minute.

Benefits

- Helps reduce tech neck soreness
- Releases rounded shoulders and back from long periods of sitting or driving
- Strengthens the upper body muscles
- Encourages full range of movement in the shoulder ball and socket joint
- Reduces the chances of long-term chronic pain or injury
- Helps release tension and stress, which is often stored and builds up in the head, neck, shoulders and back
- Keeps joints supple, mobile and loose

Top tips

- You will feel the burn! That's the lactic acid building up in the muscles under resistance. Don't forget to breathe.
- If it's too intense, take a wider, looser grip. Then progress, making it narrower and tighter, over time.

10 Second Balance Snack

Stand and balance on one leg for 10 seconds for a longer life!

Researchers have found that people who failed a 10 second balance test of standing on one foot were nearly twice as likely to die in the next decade. This is very important for us women, as we start losing our balance in midlife. The simplest snack in the book to fit into your daily routine, and one that really could make a big difference to your life as you age.

Method

1. The goal is to balance on one leg and count to 10 and repeat on the other leg.

2. To begin with, keep your hands or fingertips resting on a fixed work surface/wall/sink for support, if you're feeling unsteady.

3. As your balance improves, use less support to potentially put your hands on your hips.

Here are some targets for different age groups that you can work up to.

- Under 40: 45 seconds with eyes open, 15 seconds with eyes closed
- Age 40-49: 42 seconds open, 13 seconds closed
- Age 50-59: 41 seconds open, 8 seconds closed
- Age 60-69: 32 seconds open, 4 seconds closed
- Age 70-79: 22 seconds open, 3 seconds closed
- Age 80+ : whatever you're able to manage – aim for 10-15 seconds, with eyes open

Benefits

- Reduces the risk of falls
- Builds core strength and body alignment
- Helps maintain coordination
- Breaks up the sedentary day and helps correct any postural imbalances that can arise from just sitting
- Good for the brain
- Strengthens bones to help prevent osteopenia and osteoporosis

Next steps

- Try habit stacking. Progress by trying to brush your teeth on one leg. This ties balance on to an existing daily habit. I do this snack by default twice a day.
- Try some variations like going up on to your tiptoes, doing a few small knee bends, gazing up at the ceiling, or trying different arm positions. Try standing on one leg to put a shoe on.
- Do the Pelvic Floor Snack on page 88 at the same time, so you've ticked off two essential midlife snacks together.

Pelvic Floor Snack

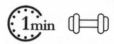

Do you leak a little urine when you sneeze, laugh or cough? You're not alone. Pelvic floor exercises are a must for everyone.

The pelvic floor muscles are a supportive sheet of muscles stretching from the tail bone at the back to the pubic bone at the front. Much like you may strengthen other muscles in your body by lifting weights, doing pelvic floor exercises (also called Kegels) is a way to keep your pelvic floor muscles strong.

These exercises are key as we age and issues can arise, commonly after childbirth and through menopause. As oestrogen levels drop at the time of the perimenopause and menopause, your pelvic floor needs your help – every day.

Method

1. Sit/lie down/stand with your feet flat on the ground and legs slightly apart.

2. Close and draw up the muscles around your back passage (as if you're trying to stop passing wind). Imagine a blueberry lodged in your back passage and hold it!

3. Then close and draw up the muscles around your urethra (as if you're trying to stop the flow of urine).

4. Hold this for a few seconds and relax. You can gradually lengthen the hold. The goal is to squeeze for 10 seconds and relax for 3 seconds, and repeat 10 times.

5. You can also try doing short squeezes where you squeeze for 1 second and relax for 2 seconds, and repeat 10 times.

6. Don't hold your breath during these exercises, simply breathe normally.

Start off small (as with everything) and gradually aim for 10 long squeezes, followed by 10 short squeezes, 3 times a day.

Benefits

- Strengthens the muscles around your bladder, bottom and vagina
- Reduces the occurrence of urinary incontinence
- Treats pelvic organ prolapse
- Makes for better sex too

Next steps

- Stack on to a strength snack. Studies are indicating that low muscle mass and strength are associated with higher rates of urinary incontinence in women, particularly those of menopausal age.

Sprint Snack

Take your fitness up a notch by adding some sprints into your walk.

When you hear the scary word 'sprint' you think of outdoor running, athletes and medals. But we can all add a small sprint into any cardio activity.

Method

1. Although this is a 1 minute snack, sprints could start at 5/10 seconds and you could repeat this snack a few times with a slower pace in between. Or you could build up to longer sprints that last 30 seconds as your stamina and fitness increase.

2. The sprints are meant to be hard, so they're quick and get you into anaerobic heart rate zones, when breathing becomes difficult. But remember, everyone is different so the intensity and pace are very individual. Start off slowly, and be careful not to overdo them.

Benefits

- Increases your cardiovascular fitness and stamina
- Burns more calories in a short amount of time

Next steps

- Make sure you cool down and stretch. Try the Standing Stretch Snack on page 147.

End of Day Stretch Snack

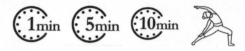

My favourite end of day stretches, based on my top yoga moves, to ease away any tension or tightness from the day.

Yoga can help manage not only the physical but also the psychological symptoms that many women experience during the transition from perimenopause to menopause.

Yoga helps with stress reduction and can improve sleep. It can help relieve menopausal symptoms, such as hot flushes, joint and muscle aches. It helps to engage the parasympathetic nervous system, to rebalance your emotions, and it can reduce meno-rage, anxiety and low mood. It's also wonderful at restoring depleted energy caused by insomnia and fatigue in midlife.

Method

If you just have 1 minute, pick 1 stretch. I usually indulge in a child's pose, as that's my ultimate favourite, but do find yours.

If you have 5 minutes, just do the first 5 stretches listed, which is the perfect daily snack-size self-care goal to commit to.

If you're feeling tight and need a little bit of extra TLC this evening, do all 10 stretches for a long self-care stretch, the perfect treat for your body and mind. (Better than a glass of wine, in my opinion!)

Treat yourself – get down on your mat/rug, set a timer or just go with the flow, with 3–5 breaths for each move.

1. **Puppy dog**: From all fours position, walk your hands forward about a palm size. Extend your bum towards the sky and let your chest and forehead melt towards the floor, with straight arms.

2. **Downward dog with hamstring pedals**: Start on your hands and knees, with your hands stacked under your shoulders and knees under your hips. Spread your hands wide and lift your tail bone/hips, drawing them towards the ceiling. Straighten your legs as best you can and alternate pressing your heels gently towards the floor. Your head should be between your arms, facing your knees, and your back should be flat.

3. **Low cobra**: Lie on your stomach with your legs straight out behind you. Place your elbows under your shoulders and your forearms on the floor as you lift your chest up off the floor. Press your hips and thighs into the floor and think about lengthening your spine while keeping your shoulders relaxed. Squeeze your glutes and lift up to feel a nice stretch in your lower back and the front of your body. (Progress to full cobra by moving your palms back towards your armpits and straightening the arms fully.)

4. **Pigeon**: Start on your hands and knees and bring your left knee forward towards your left wrist. Slide your right leg straight back. Your left heel should be close to your right hip. Elongate the spine, and gaze up, easing your right hip towards your left foot. Deepen by coming forward to rest your forearms or even your forehead on the ground, breathing deeply throughout, for up to 30 seconds each side.

5. **Child's pose**: From all fours position, knees apart, send your bum back towards your heels and lean forward to rest your forehead on the floor. Arms can be straight out in front, or next to your legs, palms facing up. Feet can be a hip width apart, or bring your toes together.

6. **Cossack stretch**: From all fours position, extend one leg out straight to the side and slowly rock back, bringing your bum to the back of the heel. Sink back and lengthen your arms or rest on your forearms; hold for up to 30 seconds each side.

7. **Cat/cow**: From all fours position, extend your tail bone/bum, arching your back and chin upwards; hold here for a few deep breaths. Then reverse this movement by tucking your tail bone under, chin to chest, rounding your back; hold and breathe into this.

8. **Butterfly stretch**: Sit on the floor with the soles of your feet pressing into each other. Root down into your legs and sitting bones. Elongate and straighten your spine, tucking your chin in towards your chest. With your exhale, fall heavy towards the floor and relax or sink a bit more deeply into the stretch. To deepen the intensity, move your feet closer in towards your hips.

9. **Lying hamstring stretch**: Lying on your back, lengthen one leg out straight up towards the ceiling. Put your hands behind your thigh and bring it towards you, holding for up to 30 seconds on each side. A belt or band looped around your foot, which you can hold, can really help facilitate this stretch.

10. **Feel Good Finish Snack**: see page 82.

Benefits

- Reduces fatigue
- Prevents muscle strain injuries
- Improves posture
- Increases muscle coordination and balance
- Helps with flexibility and mobility
- Eliminates any of the stresses from the day
- Improves your mood and reinforces positive thoughts
- Soothes any muscle tension
- Promotes better sleep

Next steps

- Stack on a breath snack or select a self-care snack from the menu.
- Stack on some journaling as an end of day ritual. If you've got 11 minutes, try the Expressive Writing Snack on page 303 and the 1 minute Dose of Vitamin G Snack on page 285.

Top tips

- Tie the moves in with your breath to get the best relaxing and de-stressing effects.
- Place a mat by your bedside or in the living room - or roll it out by your desk or workspace - as a reminder to do this exercise at the end of each day.
- Maybe light a candle and put on some soothing music.

HIIT Snack

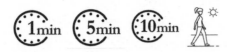

Here's 1 minute to start, then build up to 5 minutes or even 10 minutes, depending on what you fancy plus the energy and time you have available.

Don't be scared of HIIT – these moves can be high or low impact (with or without jumps), whatever pace suits you, and are still really effective.

Equipment

- A timer would help – I use free Tabata apps on my phone
- Tins, bottles or light dumbbells

Method

- **1 minute HIIT**: Pick 3 exercises from the list. The key is to simply get moving. Perfect to do a few times a day as a snack break when sitting too long. Just get up and treat yourself to this minute. Aim for 15 seconds on, 5 seconds off. But do whatever you can – even 4 seconds on, to start with, is effective – and build up from there.

- **5 minutes HIIT**: Take your pick of 5 exercises, put a timer on and do EMOM (Each Move On the Minute). Start each move on the minute and do as many seconds as you can.

- **10 minutes HIIT**: For a longer challenge, pick 10 exercises and do EMOM. Or try 30 seconds on, 30 seconds off, building up to 50 seconds on, 10 seconds off.

Choice of exercises

1. **Boxing**: March or jog while punching your arms out and holding tins or light dumbbells if you'd like to add in a weight. Vary punches forwards, upwards and sideways.

2. **High knees and rope pulls with arms (high/low impact)**: Lift your alternate knees towards your belly button and imagine pulling on a rope with your arms. These movements can either be fast or slow.

3. **Star jumps (high/low impact)**: Step one or both legs in and out, with arms meeting to clap above your head. You can do this with or without jumping.

4. **Walk, jog or sprint**: Do this on the spot.

5. **Burpees or fast step outs**: Stand with your feet a shoulder width apart. Lower yourself into a squatting position. Place your hands on the floor in front of you. Step or jump your feet back so that you are in a high plank position. (If you want to, add in a press-up!) Step or jump your feet back towards your hands and jump or straighten up to standing.

6. **Mountain climbers**: From a high plank position, alternate bringing one knee in (to your chest or opposite elbow), then back out again.

7. **Walk outs**: Stand up straight with your feet a shoulder width apart. Bend over and touch the floor with the

palms of your hands, bend your knees as much as you need. Walk your hands out, as far as you can, to a high plank position. Then walk back up to the starting position. Go fast or slow.

8. **Ice skaters**: Start by standing on one leg. Hop from side to side, switching legs, as if you were hopping over a puddle or speed skating. Swing your arms side to side, touching the opposite arm to the opposite standing leg, lowering your body down to do so. For a low-impact version do **curtsy lunges** (see page 116).

9. **Side-shuffle steps and 10 punches**: Move to one side using small, quick shuffle steps (4–10 steps, depending how much space you have) and then add 10 punches into the air. Repeat this back to the starting position.

10. **Squat jumps**: Stand with your feet a shoulder width apart and your knees pointing forwards in the same direction as your toes. Bend your knees, pressing your hips back as if you were going to sit back on a chair. Pushing through the heels, jump straight up. Land lightly with your knees slightly bent and go back into the squat position. Keep repeating and when tired just go into normal squats.

Benefits

- Better cardiovascular fitness
- More control of blood sugar levels
- Improved focus and concentration
- Boosts self-confidence
- Helps you sleep better

Next steps

- Start with a mobility snack. For example, the Daily Wake-Up Snack on page 154, or even a 3 minute Stair Snack on page 106, or a few minutes of the Feel Good Walk Snack on page 207, to warm up the body.
- Do a stretch snack after this. Ideally, the longer 10 minute End of Day Stretch Snack on page 92.
- At times of the month when you're feeling hormonal, a low-impact and/or seated version is a good idea. See the Cardio Seated Snack on page 185.

Top tips

- Pump up your favourite tunes to get you into the zone!
- HIIT snacks are perfect to tie on to an existing habit. For example, every time you boil the kettle, or when the veggies are cooking, or in between meetings or household chores!

The power of HIIT

HIIT (High-Intensity Interval Training) involves short but sweet intervals of vigorous-intensity aerobic activity. The idea is to perform an activity at a high-intensity level for a short period, followed by a recovery period.

HIIT snacks of short bursts of intense training provide the maximum release of the human growth hormone (HGH), which starts to decline once we hit our thirties, after which time we start to lose between 3 and 8 per cent of muscle per decade.

HIIT is said to be good for women in the menopause transition and can work metabolic magic in midlife. It improves insulin sensitivity and lowers fasting blood sugar levels, which is good for your overall cardiovascular and metabolic health, especially during peri/menopause when blood sugar can be harder to manage.

It can also strengthen and increase the amount of your energy-producing mitochondria. HIIT increases your stroke volume (how much blood your heart pumps per beat), improves your fat-burning capacity, and helps manage visceral (deep belly) fat, which increases during menopause. By putting a high demand on your muscles, HIIT also increases testosterone, which can help with low libido.

A major bonus of HIIT is that it's an exercise method designed to burn more calories in a shorter amount of time. In a small study of postmenopausal obese women, the women who participated in HIIT were likelier to stick with their programme and lost twice as much weight as the women assigned to an endurance programme. What's more, the HIIT group significantly changed fat mass, body mass index and fat-free mass.

Another alleged benefit of HIIT is your body's ability to stay in metabolism-boosting mode long after your workout is finished. Known as the 'afterburn effect', this process keeps you burning calories after exercise.

Shake things up with some HIIT snacks

I enjoy HIIT now and again, but don't personally believe in overdoing it. I'd much rather do strength training but mix things up by sprinkling in a short dose of HIIT once or twice a week, or even a minute a day!

The exercise routines we adopted to stay fit and healthy in our twenties to early forties no longer work the same way as we age. I also know that many people are scared of HIIT, so I always offer low-impact options for all the exercises so that all ages and abilities can benefit from it. I actually prefer low impact myself, as I find I need to be kinder to my joints more as I age. These adaptations are important during the peri/menopause when our hormones are on a roller coaster ride, and we have fluctuating symptoms. Things like lack of sleep, joint pain and vertigo can 'hiit' you hard! It's so important to listen to your body and change the intensity, frequency and duration accordingly.

You don't have to spend as much time doing these exercises. And as they include alternating intervals of quick, intense spurts with restful stages, they allow your muscles to be challenged and safely pushed to their maximum ability. Although saying that, every week I see seniors doing pretty challenging, fast-paced, low-impact HIIT bursts in my virtual workouts, and it's so inspiring!

One necessity for me is to have good music to make it more enjoyable. Boost your performance with your favourite tunes. HIIT it, DJ!

Snacks are the best for HIIT and short intervals are ideal

The best part of high-intensity interval training is that even though it's really hard, it doesn't have to be long. In fact, it's better to keep the high-intensity bursts short. When your intervals go past 60 seconds long, you can experience increases in the stress hormone cortisol. Cortisol gives you a surge of energy, so it's not necessarily a bad thing, but you don't want the levels of those stress hormones to stay elevated longer than necessary, especially during menopause, when cortisol can already be elevated.

The beauty of HIIT (high or low impact) is that it can be done anywhere, with minimal/no equipment. I like mixing up the work and rest time periods, depending on how I feel. I think the sweet spot for menopausal and older women is intervals of 20–30 seconds or less. This is the intensity people often find easiest to maintain, and actually enjoy, because psychologically you know you can do anything for 10 to 30 seconds, and it's over in no time! But there are lots of common protocols for doing short HIIT workouts, including equal amounts of effort and recovery; longer effort with shorter recovery; or short effort with full recovery. Try them out, mix it up, see what works for you.

Best Back Stretch Snack

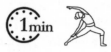

This is one of the best stretches you can do for your whole body, but especially your back and hamstrings! All you need is a wall and a desire to feel better after sitting for too long.

Method

1. Place your palms on the wall about a shoulder width apart, ideally at hip height, fingers pointing straight up.

2. Step your feet back until you're at a right angle, so your hips are directly above your knees and ankles (keeping them in alignment), and your arms are long and legs straight.

3. Keep your arms straight and let your upper body and head drop in line with your arms.

4. Hold for a minute and breathe.

Benefits

- Relieves stress and promotes relaxation
- Releases stress tension and anxiety
- Boosts mood

- Relieves back pain or sore muscles
- Increases flexibility and improves posture
- Counteracts long periods of sitting
- Makes you feel good

Next steps

- There is a more advanced version of this exercise, using a counter to lean on instead of a wall (for example, your kitchen worktop or desk). When bending to a lower level, it's harder to hold the arch in a low back while keeping the legs straight as our hamstrings and hip flexors can be too tight. I recommend starting with stretching on the wall version and then progress slowly to a counter level.
- A balance snack is also a good one to stack on to this, as well as a breath snack – think 3 Bs in 3 mins.
- For more back care, try the TLC Back Snack on page 194.

Top tips

- Think about forming an L with your body.
- If for any reason stretching on the wall does not feel good or generates pain, use your own judgement. You can either stop it altogether, or start with a shorter time and gradually increase it.

Stair Snack

3 flights of stairs 3 times a day! It's that simple! You can do it from home, work or anywhere with stairs, and ideally before or after each meal.

Just a few exercise breaks, or snacks, a day can provide significant benefits. This one really eliminates excuses for those of us convinced that we have inadequate time, expertise, income or equipment to exercise. It's so accessible and convenient. If you're working, you can stair snack on your coffee or bathroom break during the day. And rather than use the lift/escalator, climb the stairs (on your commutes too).

This is an easy way to get in some cardio, which is especially important as we are more susceptible to cardiovascular disease and type 2 diabetes through the menopause transition.

Method

1. Start off small, step by step, and build up from a few to 3 flights of stairs, 3 times a day. Build up to vigorously climbing a few flights of stairs in the morning, at lunch, and in the evening. (Go as quickly as you can, but use the guardrail for safety.)

2. To progress, take 2 stairs at a time. Add some shopping bags or a rucksack or the laundry basket as weights to progress and increase your load. It's a great way to get your housework done too – make it inefficient, with smaller laundry piles, so you have to go up the stairs 3 times!

3. Add more flights, or increase your pace, as you find it becomes easy. See how you feel – are you less out of breath?

4. Spice it up! Step 2 stairs at a time; do side steps; step up and add a high knee or glute kickback; do a squat every few stairs, or even a box-step pattern.

Benefits

- Improves cardiorespiratory health and fitness
- Increases aerobic fitness
- Boosts strength and power
- Helps control blood sugar levels, especially after a meal

Next steps

- If you have time, stack on the Lower Body Strength Snack on page 114 or the Squat Snack on page 221.
- Finish with the Standing Stretch Snack on page 147 or the Post-Workout Lower Body Stretch Snack on page 180.

Top tips

- Add a rucksack on your back when you're on your Feel Good Walk Snacks (see page 207) and find some steps to add your Stair Snack in.
- Focus on the way down as this eccentric movement may be better for you than going up.

Upper Body Strength Snack

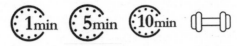

1/5/10 moves in 1/5/10 minutes to help strengthen your upper body and give you more sculpted arms.

Remember, the more muscle we have, the better our future!

Equipment

All you need are some tins, plastic bottles or weights.

Method

Select as many exercises as you have time.

1. Start by doing each move for 30 seconds, with 30 seconds rest in between.

2. As you progress, increase to doing each move for 40 seconds, with 20 seconds rest in between.

3. When you feel ready, advance to doing each move for up to 1 minute, with less or even no rest in between, i.e. doing the moves back to back.

Progress from bodyweight to light weights to heavier weights gradually, over time, as your strength increases. Correct form is essential. You can also use tempo to make the exercise harder by going slower on each rep.

If you only have 1 minute just do press-ups – the best upper body exercise!

1. **Press-ups**: Keep your back straight and your core tight; bring your chest between your hands; bend your arms at 90 degrees; progress with depth, tempo and level – you can start at a wall and then incline the surface, progressing to the floor or a box, three-quarters or full high plank position.

If you have 5 minutes, do these 5 exercises for up to 1 minute each.

1. **Press-ups**: See above.

2. **Shoulder press**: Holding a weight in each hand at shoulder height, with your palms facing away from you, keep your chest up, brace your core and keep your back straight. Lift the weights directly upwards until your arms are almost straight and they are directly above your shoulders. Return to the start position.

3. **Front to lateral raises**: Start with straight arms by your side (holding a weight in each hand), palms facing down; lift your arms up in front of you to shoulder height, then back down to your thighs; then lift your arms out to the side (to shoulder height) and down. Repeat.

4. **Dips**: Sit on an elevated surface (a bed, sofa or steps), then shuffle your body off and use your arm strength to

help you to lower and then bring yourself back up while keeping the elbows facing back behind you, your fingers facing towards your body. You can try this with legs bent or straight.

5. **Bent-over rows**: Set your spine (see the Desk Reset Snack on page 76). It's key to keep your back straight and engage your core muscles. Hinge at the hips and push them back, lowering your upper body to an angle of around 45 degrees to the floor. Row the weights towards your armpits while keeping your elbows close to the side of your body; then straighten the arms.

If you have 10 minutes, add 5 more exercises.

6. **Chest press**: Lying on the ground with knees bent, extend your arms out to the side, holding your weights, elbows bent at a 45 degree angle; exhale as you push them up so the weights end up above your chest, and then lower to the starting position. Try not to arch the middle of your back, and keep your core engaged throughout.

7. **Plank shoulder taps**: Get into a high plank position. Maintain a straight line from the back of your head to your heels; start by lifting one hand and tapping it on the opposite shoulder, without rocking your hips – imagine a drink on your back you don't want to spill. Repeat with the other hand.

8. **Biceps curl**: Straighten and bend the arms, curling your weight towards your shoulders, keeping your elbows glued to the sides of your body and palms facing away

from you. Keep your back and neck straight, core tight, and try not to swing the body.

9. **Chest flies**: On your back on the ground, with knees bent, keeping arms pretty straight, palms facing inwards; exhale as you bring your hands together above your chest; try not to arch the middle of your back, and keep your core engaged throughout.

10. **Renegade row**: From a high plank, row a weight into one side of your body, keeping elbows drawing inwards and upwards and not tilting your back; pass the weight to the other hand and repeat. Try to maintain a perfect plank throughout. Bring your knees to the ground if you get tired, or just hold a plank.

Benefits

- Strengthens shoulders, back, arms, wrists and core
- Increases muscle mass, strength and tone
- Increases bone density
- Improves posture
- Improves stability and coordination
- Reduces back, neck and shoulder pain
- Strengthens and stabilizes your joints
- Increases confidence and self-esteem
- Makes you feel strong and generally badass

Next steps

- Do the Upper Body Mobility Snack on page 163, or at least the Fitness Salutation Snack on page 124 as a warm-up before this snack.

- Stretch it out by ending with the 5 minutes Post-Workout Upper Body Stretch Snack on page 177.

Top tips

- Keep those core and stomach muscles tight – imagine drawing your belly button towards your spine.
- Keep your back straight (spine long and strong) and shoulders back and down (see the Desk Reset Snack on page 76).
- Remember to breathe throughout, using exhales during the harder/push part of the move.
- Keep going. Consistency pays off! Practice, perseverance and patience – especially with exercises like press-ups, which can take a long time as your upper body strength increases over time.
- To add some variations to the biceps curls, you could use the other exercises in the Biceps Snack on page 137.

Lower Body Strength Snack

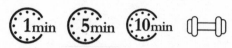

Get this done to strengthen and work every single muscle in your lower body (and your core) in just 10 minutes. Think long, lean, strong legs to keep you fit as you age.

During menopause the loss of oestrogen can lead to an increased risk of osteoporosis. When oestrogen declines, you can lose bone strength and density, and become more at risk of fractures. Strength training helps to reduce this effect.

The beauty of this workout is compound exercises. While 'isolation' exercises use just one muscle or muscle group at a time, 'compound' exercises are multi-joint movements that work several muscles or muscle groups – so you get more bang for your buck! I love compound moves as they translate to common movement patterns and work more muscles at once (both effective and time-saving).

Equipment

All you need are some tins, plastic bottles or weights, and a rucksack is always handy.

Method

1. 1/5/10 moves in 1/5/10 minutes, but if you only have 1 minute just do squats.

2. Either set a timer for 10 minutes and start each exercise on the minute, or count the repetitions of each movement, depending on how you're feeling that day. Aim for 8–12 reps for each exercise.

3. Start off using just your bodyweight and then add in weights gradually over time. Apply the principles of progressive overload to this workout. Ideally, you want to lift heavier as you get stronger – to increase muscle mass and reduce the risks of osteoporosis, plus all the other benefits of strength training, which are essential for menopause and beyond (see page 61).

4. If you reach the point where you can't go heavier, play around with the tempo of the exercises – on the way up and on the way down. The slower you go, the more time under tension for the muscles too, so tempo is a great way to progress and get stronger.

Choice of exercises

1. **Stepping**: Simply walk, jog or run on the spot to get warm. Swing your arms too.

2. **Squats:** Stand with feet just over a shoulder width apart. Visualize sitting down on an imaginary seat, keeping your knees out in line with your toes, with your weight in your heels. Come back up to standing, squeezing your glutes at the top. (As you go down and up, check you can see your toes so your knees are staying back.)

3. **Step ups**: Use a step, sturdy bench or sofa. Use your bodyweight to push through the front foot that is stepping, and squeeze your glutes as you step up. Engage your core for balance and stability.

4. **Reverse lunges**: Start by standing straight and bracing your core muscles. Take a long stride back so the front knee doesn't go over the front foot; try to bend both knees at a 90 degree angle; keep your body straight as you lower (not leaning forwards); lift the back heel up and place your weight in the heel of the front foot. Step back in and repeat on alternate sides.

5. **Glute bridges**: Lying on your back, knees bent, a hip width apart; imprint your back into the ground; exhale as you peel your back off the mat, and squeeze your glutes tight at the top of the move, lifting hips as high as you can; then inhale as you lower. Adjust feet closer to glutes or further away, to see if you feel it more in your glutes or hamstrings.

6. **Side lunges**: Imagine you're in between two panes of glass and your feet are on train tracks (toes and heels parallel and in line with each other). One leg will be straight (feel the inner thigh stretch) as you lunge your weight on to the other leg - this knee will bend in line with that toe. Repeat on alternate sides.

7. **Sumo squats**: Same tips as the squats above, but your feet will be in a much wider stance and you should feel the stretch in your inner thighs and the load on your outer thighs and glutes as you go down and up.

8. **Curtsy lunges**: Putting your weight into your front foot, step back and around with your other foot - almost

as if you're curtsying. Back straight, chest proud. Stop lunging when your back thigh is parallel to the ground. Begin to straighten your front leg, pushing up through your heel, and returning your back foot to the starting position.

9. **Bulgarian split squat**: Place the front of your back foot on an elevated surface and take a long stride so the front knee doesn't go over the front foot; try to go as low as you can when bending the knees; keep your body straight as you lower (not leaning forwards); keep your core tight; back straight and keep your bodyweight through the middle not forwards.

10. **Wall sit**: This isometric hold will burn and is a great way to lower your blood pressure. Simply sit against a wall; keep your back straight; knees bent at 90 degrees to the floor; core muscles engaged. Hold for as long as you can!

Benefits

- Builds muscle
- Burns calories
- Improves core strength
- Improves mobility
- Reduces the risk of injury
- Improves posture
- Increases balance
- Increases power and performance in daily activities
- Longevity gains

Next steps

- Start with the Lower Body Mobility Snack on page 169 to warm up the muscles.
- Try to always leave time for stretching. I recommend the Post-Workout Lower Body Stretch Snack on page 180.

Top tips

- Always engage your core; draw your belly button towards your spine.
- Keep your back fixed straight, with your spine long and strong.
- Remember to breathe throughout, using exhales during the harder part of the move (for example, as you come up from the low squat).

Core Snack

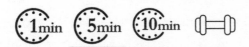

Here are 1, 5 or 10 exercises (depending on how much time you have) for you to strengthen your core, help you go about your everyday tasks with more ease, and improve your overall well-being.

Building 'ab/core' strength is about much more than physical appearance and aspiring to have a six-pack. I know myself that's a very unrealistic goal to have in midlife. I may have photos of me at forty with six-pack abs and a defined flat stomach, but I don't have that any more – and nor do I really want it! It's more important to me to have sustainable strength.

Equipment

- A timer
- A weight or dumbbell to progress

Method

Do each move for up to a minute each. Start off small and build up over time. For example:

- to begin: 30 seconds on, 30 seconds rest
- as you progress increase to: 40 seconds on, 20 seconds rest
- advanced: 1 minute on, no rest (back to back).

If you have 1 minute, just do the plank!

If you have 5 minutes, do these 5 exercises, they are the foundation for a strong core.

1. **Plank**: Lie face down with your forearms on the floor and your elbows directly beneath your shoulders. Press into your parallel forearms and rise on your toes so that only your forearms and toes touch the floor. Your body should hover a few inches off the floor, maintaining a straight line from the back of your head to your heels. Slightly tuck the pelvis under and always suck your belly button in towards your spine (imagine a rope pulling your belly up to the ceiling); take deep breaths as you hold and squeeze everything tight, including your glutes. Feet can be a hip width apart, or together is harder. You can drop to your knees for an easier version.

2. **Bicycles**: On your back, hold your head gently with your hands, elbows out. Lift your feet from the floor to a bicycle pedal motion, bringing one knee up towards your armpit and straightening the other leg while also rotating your torso. Twist so you can touch your elbow to the opposite knee as it comes up. Repeat on alternate sides.

3. **Mountain climbers**: From a high plank position, alternate bringing one knee in to your chest, then back out again.

4. **Leg raises**: Lie on your back, legs straight and together, place your hands under your bum; lift your legs all the way up towards the ceiling. Slowly lower your legs back down until they're just above the floor (without arching your middle back off the floor).

5. **Russian twist**: Sitting on the floor, lean back, bent legs on the ground (or raise them off the ground); twist your torso from side to side.

Add 5 more exercises if you have 10 minutes and if you're ready for a challenge. Perfect for when you've built up the basics. Hardcore, literally!

6. **Dead bug**: Lying on your back, with your legs raised in a tabletop position, lengthen and lower opposite arms and legs while keeping your abdominal muscles engaged.

7. **Pilates toe/heel taps**: Lie down with your knees bent and arms extended with palms facing each other. Bring your legs up to a tabletop position, one leg at a time, knees bent, thighs perpendicular to the floor. Maintain a neutral spine and avoid arching your back into the floor. Alternate lowering one foot and tapping it on the floor while the other leg remains in a tabletop position.

8. **Side plank**: Lie on one side, legs extended and stacked from hip to feet. The elbow of your arm is directly under your shoulder. Lift your hips and knees from the mat while exhaling and engaging your core tight. Your torso is in a straight line, with no sagging or bending. Hold the position for up to 30 seconds on both sides.

9. **Toe touches**: Lie on your back, with your legs extending up vertically towards the sky. Extend your arms up and crunch forwards, trying to reach up to your toes.

10. **Flutter kicks**: Lie on your back, extending your legs at a 45 degree angle or lower, without arching your back. Lift your head, shoulders and neck slightly off the ground (your arms can cradle your neck). Start elegantly kicking your legs up and down, toe pointed, alternating as you go.

Benefits

- Helps in all your functional movements and activities
- Relieves and reduces back pain
- Reduces the risk of injury
- Improves posture
- Better performance in sports or at work
- Enhances overall movement stability and coordination
- Improves your balance and reduces the risk of falls
- Helps you age well and maintain independence

Next steps

- Do the Fitness Salutation Snack on page 124 to get yourself warm and ready for this.
- If you want to do more, add on a HIIT or strength snack.
- Treat yourself by doing the End of Day Stretch Snack on page 92 after this snack for some well-deserved self-care.

Top tips

- Focus on quality over quantity: 1 minute on any of these exercises is very hard. Aim to do fewer, but properly.
- Engage your pelvic floor muscles at the same time (see the Pelvic Floor Snack on page 88).
- Contract your core muscles throughout: think belly button to spine!
- Lengthen and stretch out into a child's pose (see page 94) or cobra (see page 93), if you need to at any point. Rest, reset and restart.

Understanding your core

Your core is the centre of your body. The deep abdominal muscles help support your back, pelvis and spine, making core training an incredibly important part of any exercise regime.

Your core isn't just your toned ab muscles at the front of your body. It actually wraps around your entire torso, including muscles in your sides and back. The core muscles are like a belt that supports your spine, keeping it strong and preventing injury. So when you focus on making all of your core muscles stronger, especially the inner deep-core muscles that attach to your spine, it improves your posture, keeps you upright, and this can help you prevent some of the common neck and back pain that comes from hunching over your laptop/phone all day. Regardless of your activity outside of work, sitting at a desk or sofa for long periods of time can negatively impact your core strength, so it's vital you train it.

A strong core improves balance and stability (core work is the centre of every movement), it protects your organs, supports your strength training, boosts your power, makes everyday life easier (often called 'functional fitness' for that reason), and it helps you age well.

For more core information head to the 'menopot' section on page 12.

Fitness Salutation Snack

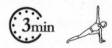

This is the best way to warm and loosen up every single joint and muscle, and a great way to alleviate the joint stiffness and pains we experience in menopause and as we age.

Essential if you sit down a lot, and ideal before any cardio or strength snacks.

Method

1. From a standing position, open your arms and reach them up as you take a big, positive inhale; then hinge at your hips to a forward fold. Place your hands in front of your feet (you can bend the knees if you need to).

2. Walk your hands out into a high plank position, then step your right foot to the side of your right hand. Sink your hips so they are parallel to the ground, and breathe into any tightness.

3. Press your left hand into the ground and bring your right hand overhead. Twist your body to the right side and bring your gaze to the lifted fingertips. Reverse the

movement and repeat on the other side. (Engage your core throughout the flow.)

4. From your plank, walk the hands back up towards your feet (with legs bent or straight) and roll up the spine to a standing position.

5. Continue for 3 minutes, or as much time as you have.

Benefits

- Improves flexibility
- Increases the range of muscle movement
- Loosens your hips
- Activates your glutes and stretches your calves, hamstrings, back and shoulders
- Wakes up the entire body from long periods of sitting
- Improves overall body strength
- Reduces the risk of injury
- Helps correct body imbalances

Next steps

- Stack on to prime you before any of your cardio or strength snacks.
- Lovely to add to your self-care snacks (see the menu of snacks and nibbles on page 269) or balance snacks too.
- To make it easier, you can start by just going into a full plank, without the foot or arm openers. Add these in as you get stronger. If you find it hard at any point, simply lower your knees to the ground.

- When doing the foot openers on each side, don't worry if your foot doesn't come all the way forward beside your hand, just bring it as far as it goes, keep your heel into the ground and sink your hips. The range and flexibility will increase, the more you practise this one.
- To progress, hold each section for longer, and really activate the muscles.

Wake-Up Stretch Snack

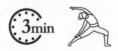

Best way to start your day! Just 3 minutes to wake your body up and treat your mind to what it deserves.

When we sleep our muscles relax, blood flow decreases, and our heart rate slows. If you are lying in the same position all night, your muscles can tighten up. It will help you start the day with a sense of calm if you've battled with poor sleep, menopausal hot flushes or night sweats. Make it a routine morning treat – a habit, just like brushing your teeth.

Method

Do what you can from the following moves. Set a timer or flow freely. Take it slow, try to hold each part of the move for a few deep breaths. Tie in your breathing with the moves, to kick-start your parasympathetic nervous system and engage your pelvic floor as you move.

1. **Forward fold**: Hang out by bending over; your chest comes towards your legs.

2. **Walk out**: Touch the floor with the palms of your hands, bending your knees as you need. Walk your hands out, as far as you can, while keeping your legs as straight as is

comfortable, to reach a plank position. Walk your hands up towards your feet and pause before unravelling the spine to standing. (See the Fitness Salutation Snack on page 124 for progressions.)

3. **Cat/cow**: From all fours position, extend your tail bone/bum, arching your back and chin upwards. Then reverse this movement by tucking your tail bone under, chin to chest, and rounding your back.

4. **Downward-facing dog**: On all fours, lift the hips up and straighten your legs, with your body resembling an upside-down V shape. You can pedal out each heel towards the ground.

5. **Puppy dog**: From all fours position, walk your hands forward about a palm size. Extend your bum towards the sky and let your chest and forehead melt towards the floor, with straight arms.

6. Add a Feel Good Hug Snack on page 80, and a Feel Good Finish Snack on page 82.

Benefits

- Great for your muscles, bones, brain and mind
- Promotes flexibility and mobility
- Helps you avoid injury
- Helps you focus throughout the day

Next steps

- Stack on a journal snack, 3 Goals for the Day Snack on page 292, and any breath snack, and you've got yourself a perfect 10 minute morning self-care ritual.

- To fire up your muscles in the morning, add on a strength snack or the Core Snack on page 119.

Top tips

- If you're short on time you can just do a quicker version - pick one move and a quick Feel Good Hug Snack (see page 80) and finish!
- If using a mat, keep it by your bedside as a handy cue.
- Try not to turn your phone on until you've got this done.

Happy Hip Snack

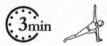

Give your hips some TLC and ease away any tightness from sitting too long. It's essential we keep them mobile. You'll greatly improve the quality of your life with happy hips.

A sedentary lifestyle can lead to stiff, tight hip flexors and hip flexor pain as excessive sitting causes the muscles to relax and deactivate. Hips also tend to carry any of your stresses. We need to do mobility exercises to get the hips feeling freer, unrestricted and moving better.

Method

3 moves in 3 minutes. Simply do each exercise for a minute. So simple but effective!

1. **Cossack rocks**: From all fours position, extend one leg out straight to the side and slowly rock forwards and back. (Like you're going into a child's pose (see page 94), rocking your bum towards the back heel and then back to all fours position.)

2. **90/90 hip openers**: Place both legs at a 90 degree angle, one in front of your body and one behind.

Windscreen-wiper the legs back and forth for up to 30 seconds. Repeat on the other side.

3. **Rocking child's pose**: From all fours position, bring your toes together and knees apart; send your bum back towards your heels (like a child's pose) and then return to the starting position. Keep rocking forwards and back.

Benefits

- Critical for healthy movement
- Loosens and strengthens hips that get tight and weak from hours of sitting
- Helps prevent lower back pain and injury
- Improves performance in other exercises
- Improves stability and strength of your hips and pelvis while walking, running, squatting, lifting, etc.
- Safeguards you against injury
- Maintains the overall health and integrity of hip joints

Next steps

- More than 95 per cent of hip fractures are caused by falling. So do this alongside your 10 Second Balance Snack on page 86 and the Gate Opener Snack on page 132.

Gate Opener Snack

This excellent exercise is one of my favourites and will not only target your balance and stability, but will work the muscles in your thighs, glutes, pelvis, hips and core too.

This standing move involves opening and closing the 'gates' of your hips.

Method

1. Pull your knee up towards your belly button, rotate the knee out and down. Then do it all in reverse to close that gate.

2. Begin with placing the foot down for a quick touch/reset after opening the gate, and progress to hovering (no touchdowns) for the whole move.

3. Keep your hips and waist forward, and body still, so the movement is isolated in the hips, driven by the leg. Stand tall, engage your core, and pull your shoulder blades down and back throughout.

4. Try to do 10 on each side. Go slow and controlled, don't rush it, for maximum benefits.

Benefits

- Reduces the risk of falls as we age and we start losing our balance in midlife
- Hits many muscles in one move
- Wakes up the hips from periods of sitting
- Helps reduce lower back and hip pain
- Works your core to keep you stable

Next steps

- This snack is an effective way to open up your hips and warm up your groin muscles before physical activities such as the HIIT snacks.
- I recommend doing this before any lower body strength snack.

_____

Top tips

- Stand by a wall or your desk/sofa (to grab on to, in case you feel a bit wobbly) and perform the exercise in front of a mirror to check your range and posture.
- Choose a spot in front of you to focus on. Keep your eyes locked on this spot while lifting and opening the leg.
- Do the Pelvic Floor Snack on page 88 at the same time.

Triceps Snack

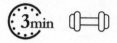 3min

Bingo wings? Tighten and strengthen the back of your arms with 3 targeted moves. To get longer, leaner and toned arms, definitely train your triceps.

Yes, having toned arms is great – especially when the sun comes out and we get our dresses and sleeveless clothing out – but I feel it's about more than just how we look, when we go through the menopause. Triceps are key players in our upper body strength when it comes to holding, carrying, pushing or pulling. Remember, your upper body strength takes time to build, it comes with practice, perseverance and patience.

Equipment

All you need are some tins, plastic bottles or weights.

Method

Do as many reps as you can in 1 minute of each of the 3 moves. The last few reps should be harder, almost to the point of failure (while maintaining perfect form, of course).

1. **Narrow press-ups**: Like a press-up (see page 110), performed against the wall, or on your knees, in

three-quarters or full floor position, but your hands are closer together and your elbows drawn in towards the side of your body.

2. **Triceps kickbacks**: Engage your core and maintain a straight spine as you hinge forward at the waist, bringing your upper body almost parallel to the floor (like RDL position on page 175). Keep your elbows in close to your body and your head in line with your spine, tucking your chin in slightly. On an exhale, engage your triceps by straightening your elbows. (Hold your upper arms still, only moving your forearms during this movement.) Pause, then inhale to return the weights to the starting position.

3. **Triceps overhead extension**: Keep your biceps and arms close to your ears; elbows stay narrow, close to each other and not flaring out, as you lower and lift the weight behind your head. Keep back and neck straight, core tight, and try not to swing the body.

Benefits

- Increases stability to your shoulders and arms
- Improves flexibility and increases range of motion
- Helps prevent injury
- Stronger upper body for your daily activities, such as carrying or pushing heavy loads
- Improves performance in upper body sports such as swimming, rowing and boxing
- Allows you to lift heavier weights in other exercises

Next steps

- Ideally stack on the Upper Body Mobility Snack on page 163 as a warm-up before this snack, or the Fitness Salutation Snack on page 124 to prep and warm up your muscles. Stretch it out by ending with the 5 minutes Post-Workout Upper Body Stretch Snack on page 177.
- Increase the weight of the second and third exercises, to progress gradually over time. If you don't want to or can't increase the weight, you can go slower with each movement – in both directions.
- Try a slower tempo with the press-ups too – down and up. The slower you go, the more time under tension for the muscles, so tempo is a great way to progress and get stronger.

Top tips

- Always engage your core. Draw your belly button towards your spine; keep your back straight and spine long and strong.
- Remember to breathe throughout, using exhales during the harder/push part of the move.

Biceps Snack

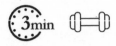

Want strong, lean, more defined, toned arms? Yes, we all do. But more importantly, do you want to stay strong, build muscle mass and be able to lift things yourself as you age? Then hello, biceps!

Biceps are essential for lifting, pulling and pushing, so they are a key feature when it comes to stronger arms.

They're key for everyday tasks such as carrying your shopping bags, lifting and pulling heavy items from a shelf, or bending down to pick something up. When it comes to building strength, you'll invariably be using your biceps for most upper body-focused exercises.

It can be really hard to see progress in your biceps, even if you're seeing big improvements in your strength. So don't be disheartened if you're not seeing major changes to your appearance straight away, you'll be enjoying a wealth of benefits that might not be visible to the naked eye.

Equipment

All you need are some tins, plastic bottles or weights.

Method

Seated or standing, grab some light weights and get curling. I've suggested three variations so you don't get bored!

1. **Wide arm curl**: Arms out to the sides at shoulder height, bend your elbows at a 90 degree angle, with your palms facing inwards; slowly extend your arms straight to sides, and then slowly bend, returning to starting position.

2. **Biceps curl**: Try to keep your elbows glued to the sides of your body, and palms facing away from you, as you bend your arms and bring the weights towards your shoulders. Release to starting position, and repeat.

3. **Hammer curl**: Same as biceps curl, but your palms are facing inwards towards each other, thumbs up. Bend the arms and release to straighten.

Benefits

- Helps get toned, shapely arms
- Builds lean muscle mass and arm strength
- Reduces potential injuries
- Helps the development of strong bones (boosts bone density)
- Protects you from fractures and injuries, should you have a fall or accident

Next steps

- Stack on the Upper Body Strength Snack on page 109 or the Triceps Snack on page 134, if you have more time. Or add on extra rounds of this snack.

- Stretch it out by ending with the 5 minutes Post-Workout Upper Body Stretch Snack on page 177 or the Feel Good Finish Snack on page 82.
- Increase weight to progress gradually over time. If you don't want to increase weight, you can go slower with each curl, on the way up and on the way down (in fact, there's great research to show the negative or eccentric/lowering part of the movement will give you amazing results). The slower you go, the more time under tension for the muscles too, so tempo is a great way to progress and get stronger.

Top tips

- Always engage your core; draw your belly button towards your spine.
- Keep your back fixed straight, with your spine long and strong. Try not to swing your body as you do these exercises.
- Remember to breathe throughout, using exhales during the harder part of the move as you curl the weights in.

Yoga Balance Snack

Three of my favourite yoga-based moves to improve your balance, work your core and correct muscular imbalances. Standing on one leg is demanding and challenging, building both inner and outer strength and resilience. Bring some balance into your life!

For a challenge, take your eyes to the left and right. This makes the balance more difficult as the vestibular system (inner ear balance mechanism) works with the visual system (the eyes and the part of the brain – the cerebellum – that controls balance). Once you master this, the next step is closing the eyes. (Attempt this by looking at an object that is still, visualize the object in your mind, then close your eyes. This visualization may enable you to stay balanced.)

Method

I've picked my top 3. Do each pose for up to 30 seconds on the left and right foot.

1. **Tree pose**: Place your hands on your hips and raise one foot high on to your left inner thigh or shin, with your hips level and squared to the front. If you feel steady,

place your hands in prayer pose in front of your heart, or stretch your arms overhead like branches reaching into the sky.

2. **Quad stretch to dancer's pose**: Standing tall, bend one knee and bring your heel towards your bottom. If steady, lean forward and press with your foot into your same-side hand, away from your body. Reach your opposite arm forward if you can, like an elegant dancer.

3. **One-legged chair pose**: Inhale and raise your arms overhead, then exhale and bend your knees so that your thighs are as nearly parallel to the floor as possible. This is the chair pose (which you can return to from the balance challenge); lift one leg off the floor and put that foot on to the supporting leg's knee for a one-legged chair pose and your hands in a prayer position.

Benefits

- Increases body awareness and proprioception through balance
- Boosts confidence and self-esteem
- Creates a strong sense of groundedness
- Prevents future injuries and falls
- Strengthens your core
- Improves posture and alignment, counteracting sitting
- Boosts your energy, focus and concentration

Next steps

- Stack this on to your Wake-Up Stretch Snack on page 127.
- Or do the Pelvic Floor Snack on page 88 at the same time.

Top tips

- I always recommend a prop (a chair or a wall) you can hold on to, to work on your balance.
- Keep your core tight and contracted, to help with balance and stability.
- It's best to leave your ego outside your practice! If your practice is dedicated and consistent, you will slowly see improvement in your ability to stay balanced.

Gentle Seated Hormones Snack

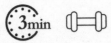

A gentle low-impact seated snack for those difficult times of the month or when your hormones are playing havoc. Restore some calm and treat yourself to some self-care movements.

As women our hormones can run havoc. It's so important to listen to your body and work with your cycle, to do what feels right for you. During menstruation, at certain times of the month, or when your periods could be all over the place with peri/menopause, it's advisable to do more restorative, low-impact and gentle exercises.

Everyone is different. Some women experience fatigue at the beginning of their period so may just want to take a rest day and do some self-care snacks. However, for me, I usually find that some light movement like this actually helps my mood and energy levels.

Here's a snack for those times when you may feel like some gentle movements, but you can even stay seated.

Equipment

- Optional light weights
- A resistance band or pair of tights

Method

6 exercises, up to 30 seconds each, back to back. Reduce the intensity or time if you're tired.

1. **Sunflowers**: Shuffle towards the edge of your chair and fold forwards, bringing your chest towards your thighs. Interlock your hands on the opposite elbows and unravel your spine as you lengthen one side of your body until you're seated upright; then roll back down to the starting position in a circular motion. Do this in both directions, visualizing you're a sunflower growing towards the sun, working with your deep breaths.

2. **Shoulder floss**: Seated version of the Shoulder Floss Snack on page 84.

3. **Seated hip circles with arm raise**: Straighten one leg and lift it off the ground; draw circles, while keeping your hips facing forwards. Circle out in both directions, and repeat with the other leg. You can hold a weight out with straight arms in front of you at the same time for a challenge.

4. **Biceps curls to press with heel raises** (with some tin cans/water bottles, if using): Keeping elbows close to your sides, lengthen the arms and then curl them towards your shoulders, and then lift the arms up towards the sky, turning palms away from you. Then bring them back to your shoulders and lengthen out to starting position. You can lift your heels off the ground during these movements also.

5. **Marching with lateral arm circles**: Simply march out the legs and get your steps in while seated, at a pace

that suits you. At the same time lift your straight arms out to the side at shoulder height and draw some small circles (with some light cans/bottles); 15 seconds in each direction.

6. **Feel-good hugs**: Seated version of the snack on page 80.

Benefits

- Elevates your mood and can actually make you feel better as exercise gives you a natural endorphin high
- Reduces pain as endorphins are a natural painkiller
- Helps manage period symptoms and may offer relief
- Can decrease PMS/perimenopause symptoms
- Eases out tension and keeps the muscles and joints working
- Ideal to do at your desk too

Next steps

- This snack is just 3 minutes. If you want to do more easy movements, stack on some stretch or mobility snacks, or some light bodyweight strength snacks.
- Light-intensity cardio is recommended to help ease period pains, fatigue, mood swings, headaches, back pain and cramps. Try low-impact HIIT (no jumps, and go at your own pace) or try a Feel Good Walk Snack (see page 207) in nature. Exposure to nature will also help boost your mood and aid with sleep if this is troublesome. See the section on nature on page 263.
- Try out some self-care snacks (see the menu of snacks and nibbles on page 269) or breath snacks to calm the body and mind further.

- If you want more seated snack options at these times of your cycle, try the band exercises in Desk/Sofa Snack on page 157, the Seated Strength Snack on page 188, the seated HIIT Snack on page 97, the Seated Stretch Snack on page 192, or the Tech Neck Stretch Snack on page 78.

Top tips

- Journaling always helps me at these times too. Try to keep a log of your cycle and symptoms.

Standing Stretch Snack

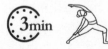

Please, please trust me! This is the best investment to reduce pains and the chances of injury.

Just 3 minutes, perfect at the end of your walk/run, before you even enter your house. Or as a post-snack cool-down. Or any time you're standing. You will thank me in the long run, it's so worth it!

Method

Ideally, you should stretch straight after every walk and always after every run – while the muscles are still warm – and hold each side for 10–30 seconds.

1. **Wall calf and hamstring stretch**: Lean your elbows against a wall or a tree; take a long stride back with one leg and keep the front leg bent. Lean and sink into the front leg and feel a lovely stretch in the back straight leg – from your bottom down to the heel. Repeat on the other side.

2. **Wide leg forward fold**: Stand with your legs wide apart and fall forwards, bringing your head towards the ground. Let the arms hang in the middle, or reach for the opposite toes.

3. **Side lunge and side stretch**: Remaining in the wide-legged position, lunge to one side, bending the knee, and lift the opposite arm up and over for a lovely side body stretch. Repeat on the other leg and side.

4. **Quad stretch**: Balance on one leg, bend the other; using the opposite hand, bring the heel towards the bottom, and try to keep the hips and knees parallel (feeling a stretch in the front thigh of the bent leg). Repeat on the other leg.

5. **Glute-leg crossover**: Holding a wall or park bench for support, lift one foot and place it on the opposite knee; sit back so you are almost seated while balancing on one leg, encouraging the bent knee to remain outwards. Repeat on the other leg.

6. **Step calf stretch**: Using a step or the kerb of the pavement, slide one heel off the edge, keeping that leg straight and encouraging the heel towards the ground to feel a lovely stretch in the calf. The other leg can have a bend in the knee. Repeat on the other side.

This is essentially your 3 minutes cool-down as it's important to bring your heart rate down. Think of it as a reward or a form of self-care.

Benefits

- Reduces the muscle and joint stiffness that can occur post-workout, known as delayed onset muscle soreness (DOMS)
- Helps the blood flow to the muscles to remove the lactic acid, which improves recovery

- Helps to relax any muscles that may have tightened up from exertion
- Reduces the risk of any injuries
- Increases the length of muscles and tendons, which in turn increases your range of motion, which then means you can move more comfortably and freely

Next steps

- If you fancy more stretching, head to your mat and try the 5 minutes Post-Workout Lower Body Stretch Snack on page 180 or the 10 minutes End of Day Stretch Snack on page 92.

Top tips

- It is helpful to focus on breathing in and out throughout the stretch.
- While it's normal to feel some tension when stretching a muscle, stretches should not cause pain. You should stop immediately, or back off the stretch until you don't feel any discomfort.
- The more you do this stretch snack, the more likely it will just become a routine habit and part of your walk or run!

Ad Break Snack

The perfect snack for the ad breaks. Or 3 minutes to get up and move every half-hour during your Netflix marathon!

This is a full body blitz of top cardio and strength moves.

Equipment

Optional weights, light dumbbells or tin cans work well.

Method

Snack on 6 exercises, up to 30 seconds each, back to back. (You can rest afterwards, when you're back to bingeing on TV. Obviously rest if you really need to, and build up to this goal.)

Always maintain proper form and technique. Mix up the tempo, going faster or even slower on the strength moves to maximize time under tension for the muscles. Enjoy the variety!

1. **Marching and boxing**: March feet (fast or slow from your seat) while punching your arms out – tins or light dumbbells are perfect for this. Vary the punches forwards, upwards, sideways.

2. **Sit and stands**: Stand up from the sofa, squeezing your glutes at the top, keeping your knees out in line with your toes, with your weight in your heels, and then come back down to touch the sofa. Keep repeating.

3. **Star jumps**: Step one or both feet in and out, with arms meeting to clap above your head – low or high impact, with or without jumps!

4. **Press-ups**: Keep your back straight and your core tight; bring your chest between your hands; bend your arms at 90 degrees; try on an incline, with hands or feet on the sofa. (The latter is harder!)

5. **Plank or mountain climbers**: Get into a plank position by maintaining a straight line from the back of your head to your heels; with hands on the sofa, draw one knee up to the chest. Keep alternating, or just hold your plank.

6. **Dips off the sofa**: Sit on the sofa edge and shuffle your body off; use your arm strength to help you to lower and then bring yourself back up, while keeping the elbows facing back behind you and fingers facing towards your body. You can try this with legs bent or straight.

Benefits

- Breaks up long periods of sitting and slouching
- Keeps the body and muscles moving and strong when we are seated
- Helps alleviate the niggles and pains we get from sitting still
- Improves functional movements to help everyday tasks
- Helps increase muscle mass
- Keeps bones strong
- Boosts your mood
- Helps control blood sugar levels (see the section on diabetes and heart health on page 20)

Next steps

- If you like this taster but want to mix it up and stay seated, do some snacks while you're watching TV – don't wait for the next ad break!
- Stack it on with the Desk/Sofa Snack on page 157, the Seated Strength Snack on page 188, the Cardio Seated Snack on page 185, the Seated Stretch Snack on page 192 or the Gentle Seated Hormones Snack on page 143.
- If you're enjoying getting up, add a 1 minute HIIT Snack on page 97, or a 3 minute Happy Hip Snack on page 130 (as our hips get tight when we sit for too long) or a Stair Snack on page 106.

Top tips

- Really focus on the muscles you're working – that mind to muscle connection is so powerful, even with bodyweight moves.
- Always engage your core and keep your back and neck straight.
- Try to move and snack on something like this after every 30 minutes of sitting (scientifically proven to be good for your long-term health).

Daily Wake-Up Snack

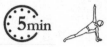

The best way to wake up sleepy muscles, joints and your whole body every morning!

Loosen your joints, release any tension, get your circulation flowing, boost your mood and feel fresh and ready for the day. A Feel Good morning ritual.

Method

Instead of hitting 'snooze' for 5 minutes, get up and treat yourself to this snack. Have a great start to your day, investing in yourself.

1. **Fitness salutation with sunflower**: See page 124 (salutation) and page 144 (sunflower) for step-by-step instructions.

2. **Warrior poses**: Choose one or a variation of these powerful standing poses, with a wide stance and outstretched arms.

   Warrior I: the front knee is bent and the hips are turned forward, with the arms raised.

Warrior II : the front knee is bent and the hips are turned to the side, with the arms parallel.

Warrior III : balancing on one foot, the standing leg is straight and the opposite leg is lifted, with the arms reaching forward.

Reverse Warrior: the legs are the same as in Warrior II, but the arms and torso reach towards the back straight leg.

3. **Squats**: Do as many bodyweight squats as you can and, for an extra opener, hold in a low yogi squat position.

4. **Press-ups**: Do as many press-ups as you can in a minute-against the wall or bed, on the floor – in a box, three-quarters, or in full press-up position.

5. **Star jumps**: Wake up the body and get the blood flowing and heart pumping with some low-impact (no jumps) or jumping jacks, being sure to clap each time so you start the day feeling like a star!

Benefits

- Relieves tension or pain from sleeping the night before
- Helps increase your blood flow
- Energizes your body
- Helps correct your posture, especially in the shoulders
- More relaxed muscles from the start of the day helps avoid tensing up and developing bad posture
- Improves your mobility
- Reduces the risk of injury
- Relieves stress

Next steps

- If you have time to do more in the morning, stack on the Wake-Up Stretch Snack on page 127, a cardio HIIT snack or a strength snack.
- Stack on a journaling snack – Daily Affirmation Snack (page 277), 3 Goals for the Day Snack (page 292), any Mindful Minute breath snack (pages 273, 279 and 283), or the 1 minute Feel Good Finish Snack (page 82) – any combination of these will just enhance how good you feel at the start of your day.

Top tips

- I suggest starting each day with this snack, but don't worry if you can't. It's just a great goal to aim for – and anytime is good, really!
- If you're using a mat, leave it by your bedside (so it also acts as a prompt or reminder).

Desk/Sofa Snack

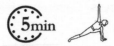

For those times when we are tied to our seats, on the sofa, or stuck in back-to-back meetings, find 5 minutes to treat yourself to this simple mobility snack.

As this snack pairs movement with resistance training it's a win-win for the muscles and joints. It's suitable for everyone and can be done seated.

Equipment

All you need is a long resistance band. A pair of old tights, or a bathrobe tie or belt, works too (keep this by your sofa/desk always).

Method

To begin with, aim for 30 seconds, then build up to the full minute on each exercise.

1. **Neck rolls and heart openers**: Circle out your head to release the neck and then place hands on shoulders; draw big circles with your elbows. Tune in with your breath as this heart opener releases the 'love hormone' oxytocin.

2. **Shoulder floss and spinal twist**: Do one shoulder floss movement (see the snack on page 84) and one spinal twist (when the band is behind your head, gently twist from left to right, then come back to centre). Repeat this duo sequence a few times.

3. **Cross-body openers**: Open out the arms diagonally in front of your chest and extend the band so you feel the resistance and a good stretch. Bring arms directly in front of you at shoulder height in between, and then change directions.

4. **Bow and arrow**: Hold your band and keep your left arm straight as you drive your right elbow back and rotate away from your extended arm, as if preparing to shoot an arrow. Then switch sides and keep alternating for up to a minute.

5. **Lat pull-down**: Hold the band with both hands, extend one arm up and keep it fixed straight by your ear, while you bend the elbow of the other arm down and out to the side, whilst squeezing the muscles in your back and shoulder blades. Alternate this on both sides.

Benefits

- Eases away soreness and tech neck
- Releases tense shoulders and rounded backs from long periods sitting
- Resistance training helps strengthen and lengthen muscles
- Encourages a full range of movement in the upper body joints
- Reduces pain or the chances of injury

- Releases tension and stress, which is often stored in the upper body
- Keeps joints loose and mobile
- Calms the body using breath combined with slow, controlled lengthening movements

Next steps

- Use as a warm-up for the Cardio Seated Snack on page 185 or the Seated Strength Snack on page 188.
- Bolt this snack on to any long meetings or Netflix sessions – seeing the resistance band will prompt you to do it, and the more you piggyback this on to your long periods sitting, the sooner it becomes a habit!

Top tips

- To progress, simply create more tension and resistance in the band by holding it tighter and with your hands closer together.

Desk
Stretch Snack

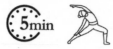

When you're stuck at your desk for hours, give yourself 5 to stretch out!

A study found that implementing stretching exercises at work also reduced anxiety and exhaustion, while increasing vitality and mental health.

Method

5 exercises to flow, breathe and stretch into. Try to hold each for 10-30 seconds.

1. **Upper body and hamstring stretch**: Seated, clasp your hands together above your head with palms facing outwards. Push your arms up, stretching upwards. Extend your legs forward, then reach towards your toes; hold wherever feels comfortable.

2. **Chest stretch**: Clasp your hands behind your back, elbows squeezing towards each other behind you; push your chest outwards and raise your chin.

3. **Angel and upper back stretch**: On your chair, place your hands behind your head and open out your elbows and chest like an angel; then place your hands on your

desk and lengthen your arms and spine; lower your head in line with your arms.

4. **Torso stretch**: Twist your upper body to one side; rest your arm on the back of your chair. Repeat on the other side.

5. **Wall angels**: Stand with your back and head pressed against a wall, knees bent. With the backs of your hands against the wall, stretch your arms straight above your head (to form a Y position) while maintaining contact with the wall; then slide your arms down towards your shoulders (like a W position). Repeat as slow controlled movements. Try not to bounce in the stretches, just hold and breathe for as long as feels comfortable. You can always release, reset and rejoin.

Benefits

- Helps you feel relaxed
- Increases your body's levels of serotonin (the hormone that can help stabilize your mood and reduce stress)
- Keeps you mobile
- Loosens up tight or sore muscles
- Aids your flexibility
- Helps you avoid injury
- Helps you focus throughout the day

Next steps

- Stack on an exercise snack to get you up and moving – a 1 minute Stair Snack on page 106, or a 10 minute Feel Good Walk Snack on page 207, or even 1 minute of the HIIT Snack on page 97.

- Or try something like the Desk/Sofa Snack on page 157 for some resistance band strength moves at your desk, or the Back Snack on page 217.
- For extra stretches, bolt on the End of Day Stretch Snack on page 92 if you're feeling tight, or the Bed Stretch Snack on page 241.

Top tips

- Never stretch through any major pain or discomfort.
- Connect the moves with your breath, and breathe deeply throughout.

Upper Body Mobility Snack

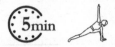

5 mobility drills, in 5 minutes, to help warm up, loosen, release, mobilize and prime your upper body and reduce aches and pains.

Method

Set up a timer for 5 minutes and enjoy the 5 moves.

1. **Spinal twists**: Place your hands behind your ears, elbows wide; twist your upper body from side to side, while hips stay facing forward.

2. **Star toe touches**: Stand in a star position and reach with one hand to touch the opposite toe. Then alternate sides.

3. **Arm circles**: Both directions, forwards and back. Singles/doubles/mix it up.

4. **Thread the needle**: On all fours, extend your right arm towards the ceiling and begin to thread it under your chest towards the ground, sliding through, aiming for your right shoulder and ear to rest on the ground. Extend the left arm overhead and breathe into this side. Then alternate sides.

5. **Lying side windmills**: Lie on your left side with your left leg extended and your right leg bent across your body at a 90 degree angle. Keep your left shoulder and hip rooted to the ground. Bring both of your arms straight out to your left side, stacked on top of each other. Rotate the right arm up and over your head while trying to touch your fingers to the ground. Allow your eyes to follow your arm as you extend it to the other side and then come back around to the starting position. Repeat on the other side.

Benefits

- Decreases soreness and joint pain
- Gives you energy and strength
- Aids recovery
- Promotes flexibility
- Increases the range of motion for increased strength potential

Next steps

- Do this before upper body strength snacks, for example, the Triceps Snack on page 134, the Biceps Snack on page 137 and the TLC Back Snack on page 194.

Top tips

- Combine some of these moves into a flow by adding in other mobility snacks.
- Log your niggles/aches/pains in your journal and see if doing snacks like this regularly helps reduce them over time.
- Seek medical advice if your pain is intense, worsens or lasts for long periods.

Shoulders Snack

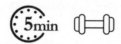

Sculpt those sexy shoulders!

Not only do they look good but strong shoulders will also help you with functional everyday activities, improve your posture, reduce pain and boost your confidence.

Equipment

- Some tins, plastic bottles or weights
- Ideally, a lighter and a heavier option (for example 3 kg and 5 kg dumbbells)

Method

5 moves in 5 minutes! If you can't, or don't want to, increase the weight, you can go slower with each movement – in both directions. The slower you go, the more time under tension for the muscles, so tempo is a great way to progress and get stronger.

1. **Shoulder press**: Holding a weight in each hand at shoulder height, with your palms facing away from you; keep your chest up, brace your core and keep your back straight. Lift the weights directly upwards until your arms

are almost straight and they are directly above your shoulders. Return to the starting position.

2. **Front to lateral raises**: Start with straight arms by your side, palms facing down; lift your arms up to the front (to shoulder height) then back down to your thighs, then to the side (to shoulder height) and down. Repeat.

3. **Upright row**: Back straight, arms straight down by your side, palms facing towards you and core tight; lead with your elbows as they draw up and out, into a hanger position at the top, with elbows at shoulder height; squeeze your back muscles and then lower your arms to the starting position.

4. **Arnold press**: Elbows together in front of you (at shoulder height), with your palms facing your forehead; twist your palms away as your lift your arms up to a straight position and then back down. Keep your core muscles engaged throughout, with your back straight and still.

5. **Plank shoulder taps**: Get into a high plank position. Maintain a straight line from the back of your head to your heels; start by lifting one hand and tapping it on the opposite shoulder, without rocking your hips – imagine a drink on your back you don't want to spill. Repeat with the other hand.

Benefits

- Stronger muscles and joints
- Improves flexibility
- Prevents injury
- Improves other strength exercises

- Protects bone density
- Increases muscle mass
- Aids carrying, pushing, lifting and overall independence
- Improves posture
- Boosts confidence

Next steps

- Be sure to warm up beforehand – stack on the Upper Body Mobility Snack on page 163 or the Fitness Salutation Snack on page 124.
- Stretch it out by ending with the 5 minutes Post-Workout Upper Body Stretch Snack on page 177.

Top tips

- Keep your core engaged, back straight. Avoid swinging your back during the exercises.
- Remember to breathe throughout, using exhales during the harder/push part of the move.
- Practice, perseverance and patience – your upper body strength takes time.

Lower Body Mobility Snack

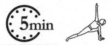

5 minutes well spent to help warm up, prep and prime, before any lower body exercises.

You could do this exercise on its own, to keep your legs nice and mobile if they are feeling tight.

Method

Set up a timer for 5 minutes and enjoy the 5 drills!

1. **March on the spot**: Literally step on the spot, fast or slow, and swing your arms.

2. **Squat to reach**: Squat down, like you're sitting on an imaginary seat behind you; as you come up to standing, reach your arms up high to the sky, perhaps lifting your heels so you're on your tiptoes too. Keep repeating for up to a minute.

3. **Standing leg swings with opposite hand to toe touches**: Swing one leg straight forwards, and try to touch its toes with the opposite hand. Keep alternating sides.

4. **Reverse lunge to high knee**: Take a long step backwards with one foot, bending your front and back

knees to an angle of 90 degrees; bring your back foot up and return to standing but try to lift that back knee high towards your belly button. Repeat on alternate sides.

5. **Froggers**: Stand with your feet spread wider than shoulder width apart. Bend at the knees; sink into a low squat and place your palms in prayer position, pushing your knees out with your elbows. To progress you can place your palms on the ground slightly in front of you and try to straighten your legs out, then bring them back to a low squat/frog position (often called the yogi squat).

Benefits

- Reduces pain and the risk of injury
- Promotes good posture
- Relieves tension associated with sedentary lifestyles (especially key for desk-workers)
- Helps prevent knots and loosens you up
- Improves all-round functional fitness performance and enhances sports performance
- Maintains joint stability to achieve the full range of motion
- Negates the shortening of muscles from other exercise or sitting too long
- Aids recovery

Next steps

- Do the Lower Body Strength Snack on page 114, the Squat Snack on page 221, the Superbrain Snack on page 287 or the Legs, Bums and Tums Snack on page 236 after this.

- Great to do before a Feel Good Walk Snack on page 207, or as part of a Grounding Snack on page 298 or a Sunshine Snack on page 305 on a nice day.

Top tips

- Like all exercises, you may feel really stiff at first, but keep practising and repeating to see how much easier mobility work gets over time.
- Tying in breath work, hand in hand with these movement flows, can also provide mental clarity that will transform your whole day and mood.
- Log your niggles, aches and pains in your journal. See if practising snacks like this regularly helps to reduce them over time.

Full Body Strength Snack

My top full body strength exercises. Get a full body blitz and get stronger in just 5 or 10 minutes a day.

This snack employs compound moves which work all your muscles and joints. Beginners start off with bodyweight and then slowly introduce weights, increasing gradually over time.

Equipment

- A selection of tins/plastic bottles/weights
- A mat and an elevated surface (sofa/bed/step/desk) for the dips

Method

For a 5 minute snack do the first 5 exercises from the list. For a 10 minute snack do all 10 exercises from the list.

1. Do each move for 30 seconds, with 30 seconds rest in between.

2. As you progress, increase to doing each move for 40 seconds, with 20 seconds rest in between.

3. When you feel ready, advance to doing each move for up to 1 minute, with less or even no rest in between, i.e. doing the moves back to back.

Don't worry if you don't have a timer, simply aim for 8–12 reps of each exercise.

1. **Squats**: Stand with feet just over a shoulder width apart. Visualize sitting down on an imaginary seat, keep your knees out in line with your toes, with your weight in your heels. Come back up to standing, squeezing your glutes at the top. (As you go down and up, check you can see your toes so your knees are staying back.)

2. **Dips**: Sit on an elevated surface (a bed, sofa or steps), then shuffle your body off and use your arm strength to help you to lower and then bring yourself back up while keeping the elbows facing back behind you and fingers facing towards you. You can try this with legs bent or straight.

3. **Reverse lunges**: Start by standing straight and bracing your core muscles. Then take a long step backwards with your left foot (with your heel off the ground). Bend your right knee until it's at a 90 degree angle, and lower your left knee towards the ground until it is also bent at a right angle. Then push back up and return to the starting position. Repeat on alternate sides.

4. **Press-ups**: Keep your back straight and your core tight; bring your chest between your hands; bend your arms at 90 degrees; progress with depth, tempo and level – you can start at a wall and then an incline surface,

progressing to the floor for a box, three-quarters or full high plank position.

5. **Plank**: From all fours on the ground, lift your knees up and maintain a straight line from the back of your head to your heels; slightly tuck the pelvis under, and always suck your belly button in towards your spine (imagine a rope pulling your belly up to the ceiling); take deep breaths as you hold and squeeze everything tight, including your glutes. Feet can be a hip width apart, or together is harder. Lower your knees to the floor for an easier option.

6. **Curl to press**: Keeping your elbows close to your sides, lengthen your arms and then curl them towards your shoulders; lift your arms up towards the sky, turning your palms away from you. Then bring them back to your shoulders and lengthen out to the starting position.

7. **Chest press**: Lying on the ground with knees bent, extend your arms out to the side, holding your weights, elbows bent at a 45 degree angle; exhale as you push them up so the weights end up above your chest, and then lower to the starting position. Try not to arch the middle of your back, and keep your core engaged throughout.

8. **Glute bridges**: Lying down, bend the legs, feet a hip width apart. Lift the hips and slowly peel each vertebra off the floor, as high as you can, squeezing your glutes at the top, and then lower back down.

9. **Bent-over row**: Keeping your back straight, engage your core muscles. Hinge at the hips and push them back, lowering your upper body to an angle of around 45 degrees to the floor. Row the weights towards your

armpits while keeping your elbows close to the side of your body; then straighten the arms.

10. **Romanian Deadlifts (RDLs)**: Begin by standing with your feet a hip width apart and knees slightly bent. Hold one weight in each hand, and place them in front of your hips, with palms facing thighs. Keeping your spine straight in a neutral position and squeezing your shoulder blades, core tight, start sending your hips back. (You want to feel this in the back of your legs, at the top, as the hips hinge and travel back – practise in front of a wall, imagining closing a car door with your bottom.) Keeping the weights close to your body, lower them down so they are in front of your shins. Maintain a neutral spine and drive through your heels to fully extend hips and knees as you come back up to standing, squeezing your glutes at the top.

Benefits

- Strengthens your full body
- Increases muscle mass
- Muscle burns more calories even at rest (muscle is more metabolically active than fat)
- Reduces the risk of osteoporosis
- Decreases the chances of injury
- Stabilizes your joints
- Aids balance, stability and coordination
- Increases confidence and self-esteem
- Includes functional moves for long-term longevity and independence
- Alleviates stress and anxiety
- Lift weights to lift your mood!

Next steps

- Always start with a mobility snack to warm up the muscles and prime the body.
- Make sure you stretch after – either combine the Post-Workout Upper and Lower Body Stretch Snacks (on pages 177 and 180) to treat yourself to some long self-care, or at a minimum do the Standing Stretch Snack (on page 147), you deserve it!

Post-Workout Upper Body Stretch Snack

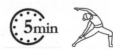

Just 5 mins of key stretches after any upper body snack to lengthen out the muscles, reduce the risk of injury, reduce any post-workout soreness, and treat your body and mind.

Static stretching after a workout is key, so stack this on after any upper body workout and hold each move for as long as possible.

Method

1. **Puppy dog**: On all fours, walk your hands forward about a palm size. Extend your bum towards the sky and let your chest and forehead melt towards the floor, with straight arms. Hold for a minute.

2. **Thread the needle**: On all fours, extend your right arm towards the ceiling and begin to thread it under your chest towards the ground, sliding through, aiming for your right shoulder and ear to rest on the ground. Extend the left arm overhead and breathe into this side for up to 30 seconds. Then do the alternate side for 30 seconds.

3. **Scorpion**: Lie down on your tummy on a mat or soft surface. Place your left hand by your armpit on the ground, your right hand straight out to the side, raise your left foot, bend at the knee and bring it over to your right side, while turning your head to look over to your left hand. Try to relax and rest your right ear to the ground. Breathe into this deep stretch for up to 30 seconds on each side.

4. **Shoulder stretch**: Straighten one arm out across your body and with the other hand draw it in towards you and look over the shoulder. Hold for up to 30 seconds on each side.

5. **Child's pose**: Kneel and sit on your knees with your knees slightly apart. Lean forward, place your arms out straight in front of you on the floor, encouraging your bottom towards your heels and, if you can, rest your forehead on the floor. Breathe deeply for a minute.

Benefits

- Reduces pain and the risk of injury
- Loosens up muscles after a workout
- Provides gradual relaxation
- Eliminates lactic acid
- Reduces the soreness you may feel later
- Keeps the muscles flexible, strong and healthy
- Helps maintain a good range of motion in the joints
- Strengthens, loosens and lengthens muscles

Next steps

- If you're working, this is the perfect snack to encourage moving when sedentary. Take this outside and combine it with the Grounding Snack on page 298 or the Sunshine Snack on page 305 for a nature boost. Check out the menu of self-care snacks and nibbles on page 269 and recovery nibbles on page 318, or stack on the TLC Back Snack on page 194 to really invest in your back and upper body.

- You could combine this upper body stretch snack with the Post-Workout Lower Body Stretch Snack on page 180 for a Full Body Stretch Snack, or just pick 'n' mix a few exercises from each, depending on how much time you have.

Top tips

- Play some relaxing music and light a candle to create a lovely calm vibe to stretch in.

Post-Workout Lower Body Stretch Snack

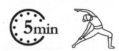

Your legs will thank you after these 5 stretches – essential after a lower body snack or perfect anytime the legs need a release. Stretch for success!

When the body cools down, the brain releases endorphins, the natural and healthy feel-good chemicals. So, after a good stretch, you'll be energized and ready to meet any challenge – let's go!

Method

Static stretching is when you hold each stretch for up to 30 seconds on each side, to really lengthen and release the muscles. Perfect if your legs are aching after a long Feel Good Walk Snack (see page 207) or a strength snack. Grab 5 mins to treat yourself.

5 moves in 5 minutes.

1. **Quad stretch**: Standing tall with your feet together, bend one knee and use your hand to pull your heel towards your bottom and keep your knees together.

2. **Hip stretch**: Kneel on one leg and bend the other leg out in front of you, with that foot flat on the floor. Keeping your back straight, slowly push your hips forward until you feel a stretch in the upper thigh of your back leg and hip.

3. **Lying/elevated hamstring stretch**: Lying or standing, lengthen one leg out straight. Raise your arms overhead; with a straight back, lean towards the leg, bringing your chest towards the thigh and reaching your hands either to your toes or shin/thigh; flex the toes towards you, and hold.

4. **Lying glute stretch**: On your back with your knees bent, cross your left foot over your right quad. Lift your right leg off the floor. Grab on to the back of your right leg and gently pull it towards your chest.

5. **Pigeon**: Start on your hands and knees and bring your left knee forward towards your left wrist. Slide your right leg straight back. Your left heel should be close to your right hip. Elongate the spine, and gaze up, easing your right hip towards your left foot. Deepen by coming forward to rest your forearms or even your forehead on the ground, breathing deeply throughout.

Benefits

- Enhances flexibility and reduces muscle tension after a workout
- Increases flexibility
- Improves blood circulation
- Eliminates lactic acid (which is produced by muscles when you work out, and can make them sore and fatigued)

- Boosts your energy
- Alleviates pain
- Increases the range of motion
- Increases muscular coordination
- Slows down the body
- Relaxes your mood, and relieves stress

Next steps

- Check out the menu of self-care snacks and nibbles on page 269 and the recovery nibbles on page 318 (for example, foam rolling, cold water therapy, or a massage or bath).
- If you want a Full Body Stretch Snack (after a full body workout) you can combine this lower body stretch snack with the Post-Workout Upper Body Stretch Snack on page 177. And if you're short on time, just pick 'n' mix a few from each snack, depending on how much time you have. It's flexible, just like you will be!
- Engage your pelvic floor and tummy muscles while you're doing these exercises – see the Pelvic Floor Snack on page 88.

Seated Circulation Snack

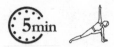

The perfect snack for your desk or sofa, to boost circulation, keep the blood flowing, loosen up your joints and warm up your muscles.

This snack is especially beneficial when you're feeling cold or craving some easy movements.

Method

Sit nice and straight and set a timer for 5 minutes. There are 10 moves, so aim for 30 seconds of each exercise. Change the direction of the movement every 15 seconds (this coordination will also help keep your brain fit).

1. **Neck rolls**: Imagine a clock right in front of you; using your nose, draw a circle around that clock – in both directions.

2. **Shoulder circles**: Lift your shoulders up and roll them back in a large circular motion. Then repeat forwards.

3. **Arm circles**: Circle your arms forwards and backwards.

4. **Left leg circle**: Lift your leg and draw circles while keeping your hips still – in both directions.

5. **Right leg circle**: Lift your leg and draw circles while keeping your hips still – in both directions.

6. **Spinal twists**: Place your hands behind your ears, elbows wide; twist your upper body from side to side.

7. **Ankle and wrist circles**: Lift each leg in turn and circle out the ankles and wrists.

8. **Point and flex**: Feet lifted or down, straighten your legs and point your toes away and stretch out your fingers; then flex toes towards you and hands make a fist.

9. **Heel raises and toe raises**: Lift your heels and press down on your tiptoes; then press heels down and lift your toes.

10. **March on the spot**: Literally step on the spot.

Benefits

- Improves joint mobility
- Encourages the full range of movement and lubricates the joints
- Warms and loosens up muscles
- Breaks up long periods of sitting
- Can reduce aches and pains

Next steps

- If you have more time, stack this with the Seated Strength Snack on page 188.
- And/or stack this with the Seated Stretch Snack on page 192.

Cardio
Seated Snack

Yes, you can even get a bit of HIIT when seated, for the times when you're stuck at your desk or on the sofa, or simply want to take things easier. This will help you keep the joints mobile, the muscles activated, and work your heart, lungs and respiratory system – together with a nice release of endorphins, all in just 5 minutes.

Here are 5 of the top moves from my free Feel Good YouTube workouts with my mother-in-law. Perfect if you're stuck behind your desk (on virtual meetings) or maybe watching TV too long, or recovering from an injury, or not able to stand. Also if it's your time of the month, or you're battling with hormones or just feeling tired. This is a great snack for seniors or people who are less mobile.

All these moves are low impact (without jumps) and suitable for all ages.

Equipment

- A timer
- Some tin cans or light weights (you could even buy ankle or wrist weights)

Method

EMOM: Start each move on the minute, and do as many seconds as you can. Build up your stamina gradually. Vary the pace, to match your energy.

1. **Swimming**: Visualize doing some breaststroke or forwards/backwards crawl, with some marching on the spot.

2. **Star jumps**: Step one or both feet in and out, with arms meeting to clap above your head.

3. **High knees with rope pulls**: Lift one knee at a time up towards your chest while imagining pulling a rope with alternate arms.

4. **Boxing**: Punch all your worries away while walking, jogging or sprinting on the spot from your seat.

5. **Skipping**: Hold an imaginary rope with your arms, circling and jumping or stepping with single or both feet as the rope swings.

Benefits

- Burns calories from a chair
- Breaks up long periods of sitting
- Works the heart, lungs and respiratory system
- Controls blood sugar levels
- Encourages joint stability, range of motion and mobility
- Strengthens the bones, muscles and brain
- Increases flexibility and strength
- Increases coordination
- Increases circulation

- Improves posture and balance
- Boosts your mental health

Next steps

- Start with a Desk/Sofa Snack on page 157 using a resistance band, or a Seated Circulation Snack on page 183.
- If you have more time, add on the Seated Strength Snack on page 188.
- Finish with the Seated Stretch Snack on page 192.

Top tips

- Get your family members to join in.
- Listen to your body, rest when you need to, and some days may be easier than others.
- See how your stamina and fitness change over time; journal your progress.

Seated Strength Snack

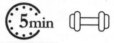

You can get strong even when you're seated! There's no excuse not to build muscle and future-proof our bodies.

This is perfect to do from your sofa/desk, or when it's your time of the month or you're battling with hormones. Or even if you've just had a heavy meal and you need to sit. Strength training is an antidepressant and will help combat that sluggish feeling we get when we are seated.

Equipment

All you need are some weights – tin cans, plastic bottles or dumbbells.

Method

Do as many reps as you can on each move, each minute. Make sure you focus on proper form and technique, especially with the combination moves. Go slowly up and down on each move to increase the time under tension for the muscles – and for great results.

A good gauge that you're using the right weight is when the last few reps feel challenging. But you don't always have to go heavier; you can do more reps, or take less rest, or go at a slower tempo.

1. **Biceps curls to shoulder press with heel raises**: Keeping your elbows close to your sides, lengthen your arms (with some cans/water bottles) and then curl them towards your shoulders; lift your arms up towards the sky, turning your palms away from you. Then bring them back to your shoulders and lengthen out to starting position. You can lift your heels off the ground during these movements too.

2. **Shoulder press with alternate leg extensions**: Holding a weight in both hands at shoulder height, with your palms facing away from you, lift the weights directly upwards until your arms are almost straight and they are directly above your shoulders. At the same time, alternate lifting one leg off the ground and holding it straight, to activate your thigh/quad muscles.

3. **Overhead triceps extensions**: Bend your elbows, hands clasped over the weight you're using, and lower the weight behind your head as far as you can, keeping your back upright, elbows close to your head and core engaged. Then, at the lowest point, straighten your elbows and extend the weight back overhead.

    Or triceps **dips**: off your chair (see the Upper Body Strength Snack on page 109).

4. **Front and lateral raises**: Arms straight, palms facing down, holding some light weights. Lift and lower your arms to the front (to shoulder height); then lift and lower to the side (to shoulder height). Repeat.

5. **Chest press**: Bend your arms out to the side, holding your weights at right angles; exhale as you push them inwards, almost like you're going to squeeze your elbows together in front of your chest.

Refer to the Upper Body Strength Snack on page 109 for any reminders of form and technique.

Benefits

- Activates the muscles and keeps them strong at times when we are seated (rather than doing nothing)
- Helps alleviate the niggles and pains we get from sitting still
- Increases muscle mass, strength and tone
- Increases bone density
- Helps control blood sugar levels
- Improves posture
- Helps with functional movements and everyday tasks
- Improves stability and coordination
- Helps prevent injuries
- Reduces back, neck and shoulder pain
- Stabilizes your joints
- Boosts and supports other exercises
- Increases confidence and self-esteem
- Boosts your mood

Next steps

- If you like this taster and want to do more but stay seated, stack this on to the Desk/Sofa Snack on page 157, the Seated Circulation Snack on page 183, the Cardio Seated Snack on page 185, the Seated Stretch

Snack on page 192 or the Gentle Seated Hormones Snack on page 143.

Top tips

- Really focus on the muscles you're working – that mind to muscle connection is so powerful.
- Always engage your core and keep your back and neck straight.
- Although this is good to do when seated, always try to stand and move after every 30 minutes of sitting – even if it's only for a few minutes. This is scientifically backed to be good for your long-term health.

Seated Stretch Snack

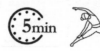

Don't just sit, stretch!

If you are sitting for too long, at least treat yourself to these quick and easy stretches to compensate.

Method

Do both sides, left and right. Hold for 30 seconds on each move, or 5-7 deep breaths, then switch sides.

1. **Upper body and hamstring stretch**: Extend one leg out straight, with the heel on the ground; reach your arms up to lengthen your spine; reach forward as far as you can and place your hands by your toes/front of your leg and hold.

2. **Side reach**: Simply raise one arm up and over your head and reach towards the opposite direction. You can loop the hand of the other arm behind your back/chair for a deeper release.

3. **Glute stretch**: Place one foot on the opposite knee and encourage the elevated knee out as much as feels good.

4. **Knee hug stretch**: Lift and bend one leg and simply hug the knee in towards your chest, maybe adding in some ankle rotations too.

5. **Triceps stretch**: Bend the arm and bring your left elbow straight up by grabbing your left elbow with your right hand. With light pressure, pull your left elbow back towards your head and almost behind it.

Benefits

- Fights tension
- May help reduce some soreness or tightness
- Improves blood flow
- Keeps your joints active and lubricated
- Encourages circulation
- Improves flexibility
- Helps with stress reduction
- Improves your mood

Next steps

- I'd tie on my 1 minute Desk Reset Snack on page 76 regularly. Add the 5 minutes seated Tech Neck Stretch Snack on page 78 too, while you're seated.
- Add on a breath snack to soothe the mind and relax you further.

TLC Back Snack

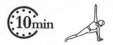

Here's a longer treat for your back – some real, well-deserved TLC. Back pain is a common complaint of women transitioning through menopause. If that's you, treat your back to this!

If you're sore, remember not to work through pain, just do what your body allows. Muscles can feel tight, and it can take time and patience to increase flexibility and enjoy a release (especially when you tie it in with your breath). But don't continue if you experience any excruciating pain – always consult a medical professional.

Method

10 exercises, up to 1 minute each. Set a timer and go with the flow!

1. **Cat/cow**: From all fours, extend your tail bone/bum, arching your back and chin upwards; then reverse this movement by tucking your tail bone/bum under, chin to chest, rounding your back.

2. **Thread the needle**: On all fours, extend your right arm towards the ceiling and begin to thread it under your chest towards the ground, sliding through, aiming for your right shoulder and ear to rest on the ground.

Extend the left arm overhead and breathe into this side. Then alternate sides.

3. **Superwoman**: Lie on the floor facedown, with your legs straight and arms extended in front. Keeping your head neutral and looking down, lift your arms and legs a few inches off the floor. Engage your glutes, your core, and lift your belly button off the floor to contract your abs. Like you're a Superwoman flying in the air. Hold for a few seconds, then lower and repeat.

4. **Angels**: Start lying on your back, with your knees bent and your feet flat on the ground, your arms out to your sides and your elbows bent at a 90 degree angle. Slowly slide your arms up over your head while keeping your elbows and wrists flat on the ground. Lower and repeat. (See the Desk Stretch Snack on page 160 for step-by-step instructions on how to do wall angels.)

5. **Lying side windmills**: Lie on your left side with your left leg extended and your right leg bent across your body at a 90 degree angle. Keep your left shoulder and hip rooted to the ground. Bring both of your arms straight out to your left side, stacked on top of each other. Rotate the right arm up and over your head while trying to touch your fingers to the ground. Allow your eyes to follow your arm as you extend it to the other side and then come back around to the starting position. Repeat on the other side.

6. **Dead bug**: Lying on your back, with your legs raised in a tabletop position, lengthen and lower opposite arms and legs while keeping your abdominal muscles engaged and back flat into the floor (not arching).

7. **Lower back stretch**: Lying on your back, bring your arms out to the sides with the palms facing down in a T position. Bend the right knee and pull it to twist over to the left side of your body. Look at the right finger tips, keeping shoulders grounded. Repeat on the other side.

8. **Lying Feel Good hug**: On your back, simply hug your knees into your chest and wrap your arms around your shins. Add some rocks from side to side, or draw some circles with the knees, to massage the lower back.

9. **Child's pose with reaches**: On all fours, send your bum back towards your heels and lean forward to rest your forehead on the floor. With arms straight out in front, reach both arms over to the left side; hold and then repeat on the right side.

10. **Forward fold release**: Stand with your legs a hip width apart and fall forward, bringing your head towards the ground like a rag doll. Grab opposite elbows and sway from side to side. Slowly unravel, vertebra by vertebra, to a standing position.

Finish with the Feel Good Finish Snack on page 82.

Benefits

- Counteracts long periods of sitting
- Relieves stiffness in your back
- Helps reduce rounding of the spine (kyphosis)
- Strengthens and engages muscles and joints
- Improves posture
- Relaxes any tension
- Reduces pain in your back, neck, shoulders and glutes

- Increases flexibility
- A form of self-care

Next steps

- This is a great one to stack on after the Back Snack on page 217, once a week.
- A breath snack coupled with this would be a great idea. It will help you focus on your breathing and get you centred and ready to mobilize.

Top tips

- Keep your core muscles engaged through all the exercises to protect your back – imagine your belly button being sucked in towards your spine.
- I love Self-care Sundays, so maybe do this snack, or the End of Day Stretch Snack on page 92, as a weekly treat to combine moving, dynamic stretches and slow, static stretches. Add on something from the menu of self-care snacks and nibbles on page 269 too.

Full Body Mobility Snack

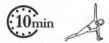

One of the best forms of self-care and a key way to future-proof your health: 10 essential dynamic movements to flow through in just 10 minutes. Flexibility or mobility training is an important dimension you must incorporate into your training, whether you're a beginner or more advanced.

Our flexibility and mobility decrease with age. Modern-day sedentary lifestyles and the prolonged use of technology are major contributors to decreasing our mobility.

For example, have you ever had to ask for help from a family member or friend when putting your arms through the sleeves of a jacket? Or have you ever struggled to simply get up and out of bed in the morning?

Alternatively, have you ever been unable to perform a strength training exercise (like a squat or a deadlift) due to poor range of movement? Has your poor flexibility held back your strength gains? Do you adjust your movement patterns to compensate for poor mobility and joint range? I think many of us women will say yes to these examples. That's why mobility is key! It's one of the best self-investments we can make!

Method

10 moves in 10 minutes. Put the timer on and take rests when you need to. Breathe deeply to release any areas of tension.

1. **Sunflowers**: From standing, fold forwards, bringing your chest and upper body towards your thighs like a rag doll. Interlock your hands on the opposite elbows and unravel your spine as you lengthen one side of your body until you're standing up straight; roll back down the other side to the starting position in a circular motion. Do this in both directions, visualizing you're a sunflower growing towards the sun, working with your deep breaths. Add in a Fitness Salutation Snack on page 124.

2. **Shoulder floss and spinal twist**: Do one floss movement (see the Shoulder Floss Snack on page 84) and one twist (see the Upper Body Mobility Snack on page 163) and repeat this dual sequence a few times.

3. **Thread the needle**: On all fours, extend your right arm towards the ceiling and begin to thread it under your chest towards the ground, sliding through, aiming for your right shoulder and ear to rest on the ground. Extend the left arm overhead and breathe into this side. Then alternate sides.

4. **Cossack rocks**: From all fours, bring one leg out to the side. Rock back and flex your hips until a stretch is felt along the straight leg groin and inner thigh. Rock forward to the starting position. Repeat on the other side.

5. **Scorpions**: Lie down on your tummy on a mat or soft surface. Place your left hand by your armpit on

the ground, your right hand straight out to the side, raise your left foot, bend at the knee and bring it over to your right side, while turning your head to look over to your left hand. Try to relax and rest your right ear to the ground. Breathe into this deep stretch.

6. **Lying side windmills**: Lie on your left side with your left leg extended and your right leg bent across your body at a 90 degree angle. Keep your left shoulder and hip rooted to the ground. Bring both of your arms straight out to your left side, stacked on top of each other. Rotate the right arm up and over your head while trying to touch your fingers to the ground. Allow your eyes to follow your arm as you extend it to the other side and then come back around to the starting position. Repeat on the other side.

7. **Frog rockers**: On all fours shift your weight forward on to your hands. Move your knees out to the sides, keeping them in line with your hips. Keep your knees bent and your ankles behind you, in line with your knees. Turn your toes out to the sides like a frog. With bent or long arms on the floor, sit back into your hips to deepen the pose and rock forwards and back.

8. **Hip flexor rock back to hamstring**: Kneel on the floor and place one bent leg with a large stride in front of you. Keeping your body tall, tilt your pelvis and push your hips forward evenly until you feel a stretch in the front of the thigh of your back leg. Next, transfer your weight backwards by taking your buttocks towards your back foot as you straighten your front knee and lift your toes, flexing towards you. You will feel a stretch in the back of the thigh of your front leg.

9. **90-90 hip rotations**: Place both legs at a 90 degree angle, one in front of your body and one behind. Twist from side to side slowly, keeping your waist facing front and feeling the movement in the hips.

10. **Yoga flow**: Start with all fours cat/cow by extending your tail bone/bum, arching your back and chin upwards; then reverse this movement by tucking your tail bone under, chin to chest, and rounding your back. Then flow into downward dog by lifting your tail bone/hips, drawing them towards the ceiling. Straighten your legs as best you can and alternate pressing your heels gently towards the floor. Then go into a plank position and maintain a straight line from the back of your head to your heels; slightly tuck the pelvis under and always suck your belly button in towards your spine (imagine a rope pulling your belly up to the ceiling). Straight into a cobra by bringing your body down on to your tummy; bend your elbows straight back and hug them into your sides; lift your chest off the floor. Then relax back into child's pose by bringing your bum to your heels, with arms extended out in front or palms facing up by your feet.

Benefits

- Improves pain
- Moves joints through the full range of motion
- Freedom of movement
- Improves joint flexibility
- Improves circulation
- Decreases the risk of injury
- Reduces muscle aches, tension and soreness
- Improves posture

- Improves movement efficiency
- Relieves menopausal joint pain
- Reduces the risk of osteoarthritis
- Better mobility as we age

Next steps

- Stack on a Full Body Strength Snack on page 172.
- Or stack on the HIIT Snack on page 97.

Top tips

- Go slow and enjoy feeling the full range of movement.
- Breathe deeply with the flow - great for calming the mind and releasing any mental tension too.
- Just go as far as you can through each movement - you may feel tighter one day, or the move may feel harder - so go with the flow. Do what your body allows, and be grateful.

Move after meals

Our modern diets are full of sweet and starchy foods (even your first meal of the day, breakfast) which are highly addictive. This is because of the pleasure hit of dopamine released in our brain when we consume them. But because starches and sugars turn to glucose during digestion, they lead to a glucose spike. The body's natural response to a glucose spike is to release the hormone insulin, which takes that glucose out of the blood and stores it in our liver, muscles and as fat for future use. Not only is this one of the ways we get fatter but, unfortunately, these spikes can harm both our physical and our mental health.

I have personally been fascinated by fluctuations in my blood sugar as I have suffered from blood sugar spikes, dips and dives since my twenties, which led to crashes where I was so famished that I would get dizzy, weak and even on several occasions passed out. Not only does this blood sugar roller coaster leave you feeling tired, low, tormented by cravings and insatiable hunger, but it also triggers a state of chronic inflammation, which accelerates the ageing process and can leave you vulnerable to disease. It can even make menopausal symptoms worse by affecting hormone levels, and in the long term this inflammation can increase your risk of developing diseases such as type 2 diabetes and Alzheimer's. I have always worried about both, as diabetes is so prevalent on my mum's side of the family, as well as Alzheimer's after we lost my grandmother to it. However, I have definitely felt better since starting my fitness journey, and especially when I tend to do some physical activity after my meals and since I started eating more protein in my diet.

It is great to see much more awareness around this subject recently. I have worn a continuous blood glucose monitor (like diabetics often use) which provides personalized nutrition information. For example, companies like ZOE are able to identify the foods which supposedly can damage your health, and provide recommendations on foods to help balance your blood sugar. I have seen at first hand the impact of movement after meals on my own blood sugar levels and how it helps flatten out the curves and prevent spikes, which has such a big impact on my concentration, mood, energy and hunger levels. To be honest, it's also made a huge difference to my perimenopausal symptoms, with fewer mood swings, less brain fog, less fatigue, better sleep and fewer outbursts of irrational anxiety.

Moving after meals actually originates from Ayurveda, the old traditional Indian custom of 100 steps after a meal. Shatpavali (*shat* means '100' and *pavali* means 'walk') is the ideal way to aid digestion, improve metabolism, relieve that post-meal laziness and food coma, as well as improving your overall well-being.

Nowadays, the American Diabetes Association officially recommends walking to lower blood sugar levels and reduce your overall risk of developing type 2 diabetes. It's almost like free medication for anyone who has diabetes, as it helps lower one's blood sugar naturally. Exercise like walking also increases insulin sensitivity, which means it allows the body to use glucose more effectively, thus lowering blood sugar levels and reducing the harmful spikes. Even among those who do not have diabetes, exposure to chronic high levels of blood sugar can increase the risk of heart disease and type 2 diabetes down the road.

Most advice is that walking for even 10 minutes (or 1,000 steps) after meals helps you digest your food, reduce your weight and sleep better. It lowers blood sugar (great for those with diabetes), speeds up metabolism and improves blood circulation. But one 2022 study published in the journal *Sports Medicine* showed specifically that just 2 minutes of walking after eating can help lower blood sugar. Even the shortest of walks can make a difference. So in essence, getting up and moving after you eat, even if it's only for two minutes, can help control blood sugar levels.

When I was on Sky News on Christmas Day 2020, I advised people to move and go for a Feel Good walk after their Christmas lunch. But we need to heed that advice after every meal, not just do this once a year or after the Sunday roast. Avoid slumping straight on to the sofa or sitting at your desk or remaining at the table, if you can, as being sedentary after eating is more likely to cause a spike in your blood sugar. Plan your dog walks, shopping trips, errands, popping to the bank or post box, watering the garden after meals. A lap around the block is not only great for blood sugar control but it's a great way to connect with your loved ones. And you'll reduce bloating, regulate your blood pressure and enjoy all the other benefits (see the Feel Good Walk Snack on page 207).

For the biggest health benefits, aim to move within 60 to 90 minutes after you finish a meal as this is when blood sugar levels tend to peak. So set a timer within this important window after each meal to remind yourself!

If you're chained to your desk or if you simply can't get a walk in, even just standing helps too. Standing requires your body to activate more muscles than when sitting or lying down. These muscles seek energy from the food you have just eaten and help take the sugar out of your bloodstream and flatten the glucose spike. It's actually perfect to tidy the kitchen straight after meals – let's look at housework, washing the dishes, mopping and hoovering as a positive! Perhaps you could add your press-ups (see the Upper Body Strength Snack on page 109) or squats (see the Squat Snack on page 221) to this. Do a Stair Snack on page 106 and run up and down a few flights of stairs, or simply play with the children or grandchildren!

Strength training is particularly effective as every time a muscle contracts, glucose is burned up, so we can help flatten our blood sugar level after a meal. Resistance training has been shown to decrease the glucose spike by up to 30 per cent, and the size of further spikes in the following 24 hours by up to 35 per cent, helping to keep the level of sugar in the bloodstream more steady throughout the day.

Pick any strength snack. The more times and the harder a muscle contracts and is activated, the more excess glucose will be mopped up from your bloodstream from your last meal.

If you can't stand up for any reason, then pick one of the seated snacks. They will still work some muscles to help soak up excess glucose. That handy weight (dumbbell or plastic bottle) next to your sofa will be a good cue for the Desk/Sofa Snack on page 157. I've even heard that simple calf raises work – lifting your heels up off the floor for 10 minutes after a meal – which are perfect if you're in a restaurant with other people. They won't even know you're doing them!

Feel Good Walk Snack

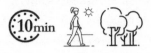

Go for a brisk walk for 11 minutes a day to reduce your risk of early death and disease. You can even break this up into shorter bite-size amounts — walk snacks.

Head out and just start walking! Expose yourself to nature, if you can. Build up to a brisk pace where you are getting warmer, slightly out of breath but able to maintain a conversation. This is moderate-intensity cardio.

If you're struggling with your sleep, going for a walk snack in the morning (ideally within 2 hours of waking up) and getting that exposure to day and sunlight really helps your body's natural circadian rhythm.

Walking is also pelvic floor friendly. Walking is a safe and proven low-impact method for strengthening your pelvic floor muscles. The pelvic floor muscles can be affected during menopause as falling oestrogen can affect our muscle strength, which can result in several symptoms and problems as we get older (including leaking when coughing or sneezing, urinary incontinence, vaginal dryness and irritation, pelvic pain and discomfort during intercourse, pelvic floor or pelvic organ prolapse).

Method

Posture is important. Try to hold your chin parallel to the ground, push your shoulder blades down your straight back and roll your stomach slightly inwards as though tucking it under your ribcage. Think about trying to roll through your foot, heel-to-toe, as you take each step.

Benefits

- Improves sleep
- Regulates hunger
- Boosts mood and releases serotonin (great if you suffer from SAD in the winter months) and feel-good endorphins
- Boosts your metabolism
- Improves energy
- Banishes brain fog, especially outside in nature
- Boosts focus, creativity and outlook
- Helps control blood sugar levels (see the 'Move after meals' section on page 203)
- Can reduce anxiety or feeling overwhelmed

Next steps

- **Go faster**: Add in short bursts at a faster pace for between 30 seconds and 2 minutes at a time. Everyone's pace is different, so just alternate hard, fast walking (when talking feels difficult) with easy, moderate walking (when you can talk comfortably). This will keep your walks more interesting and challenge you. See the Sprint Snack on page 90.

- **Go heavier**: Carry a rucksack (increase the weight you're carrying gradually over time), purchase some ankle weights or carry some dumbbells or heavy water bottles to power up your walks.
- **Go on a new route**: Find some steps or hills to challenge yourself. See the Stair Snack on page 106.
- **Throw in a strength snack**: Do this while you're on your Feel Good walk, or sprinkle in some lunges, squats or dips and press-ups on a park bench.

Feel Good walks

My favourite form of cardio is walking, outdoors, surrounded by nature. I call them 'Feel Good walks' because they always make me feel good. Walking is so underrated but one of the most effective ways to improve your physical and mental health. The best part is it's free, and it can be done almost anywhere.

Walking has helped me to lose excess fat and maintain a healthy weight, and it's my instant mood booster. I have had some of my best and most creative ideas over the last few years while walking. It has also been a magical tool in banishing brain fog and alleviating any bouts of anxiety I have experienced in my perimenopause. If I've had a squabble with one of my kids, or if I'm feeling anxious about my workload or the pace of life, walking helps me to just step away, clear my mind and release that anger, so I'm a better person when I walk back in the door. Literally walking away from my troubles! I always feel better after a walk, even a quick walk snack. It's like free therapy.

10 incredible benefits of walking

1. **Increased heart and lung fitness**: Walking for an average of 30 minutes or more a day can lower the risk of heart disease and stroke by 35 per cent. This is particularly important as our risks increase in midlife.

2. **Boosts longevity**: And can cut your risk of dying from any cause.

3. **Lowers blood sugar levels and helps manage diabetes**: A walk of 30 minutes a day can lower the risk of type 2 diabetes by 40 per cent – and you can break this up into shorter duration walk snacks!

4. **Eases and alleviates joint and muscular pain or stiffness**: All common menopausal symptoms.

5. **Stronger bones and improved balance**: Both of which we start losing in midlife.

6. **Increased muscle strength and endurance**: Key to ageing well.

7. **Helps you maintain a healthy weight**: Or lose weight, and reduces body fat.

8. **Boosts your brain**: And also your immune system.

9. **Can help beat depression and stress**: Releases endorphins and has massive mental health benefits.

10. **Improves your sleep**: Essential for mental and physical well-being.

Backed by science

Researchers at the University of Leicester have previously found that as little as 10 minutes of brisk walking each day can contribute to a longer life. These individuals had a life expectancy up to 20 years longer than their slower-walking peers. Public Health England also published a report in 2017 on the health benefits of 10 minutes a day of brisk walking in midlife.

A body of evidence including a 2016 paper from the American Heart Association links sedentary lifestyles to an increased risk of diabetes, dementia and death from heart disease. But studies show that even a 5 minute walk every half-hour was able to offset a lot of the harms of sitting. This is a game changer for people working from home and stuck in endless virtual meetings (especially since the pandemic), a common feature of the increase in sedentary lifestyles.

Latest studies show even 3 minutes walking every half-hour could help people with type 1 diabetes manage blood sugar levels. I spoke to the lead researcher of this ground-breaking trial, Dr Matthew Campbell at the University of Sunderland, which was funded by Diabetes UK, and it was fascinating to hear that what they term 'activity snacking' helps people with type 1 diabetes manage their blood sugar levels. The research revealed for the first time that short breaks from sitting time can help people with type 1 diabetes to spend more time with their blood sugar levels in target range.

Previous research has shown that breaking up periods of sitting with short, frequent walks can help people with type 2 diabetes reduce their blood sugar levels and their risk of complications. This is because being active can increase the amount of glucose (sugar) used by muscles and can help the body to use insulin more effectively. Up till now we haven't known if people with type 1 diabetes could see the same profound benefits.

I think this research is important for everyone, as we are starting to become more interested in and aware of the impact of blood sugar levels on our health, and this could help anyone manage them better.

Dr Campbell shared another important finding with me. He said, 'Importantly, this strategy also does not seem to increase the risk of potentially dangerous blood glucose lows or hypos, which are a common occurrence with more trad-itional types of physical activity and exercise.' This is great news that blood sugar levels will be more balanced with the exercise snacking approach. Avoiding the roller coaster ride of glucose spikes and dips will help people feel better, and it is much healthier in the long run.

What is amazing is that breaking up prolonged sitting with short bursts of activity is something that everyone can do, irrespective of whether they currently exercise or not. Simply set a timer to take regular breaks from sitting! For some people, this could be an important stepping stone towards more regular physical activity or exercise, whereas for others, it can be a cost-free and acceptable intervention to help manage their blood glucose levels and reduce the risk of future complications.

One of the best ways to manage your blood sugar levels and combine this with the magic of walking is to move after meals (see the section on page 203).

Walking just 11 minutes a day could prevent 10 per cent of early deaths

A 2023 report from the *British Journal of Sports Medicine* advocates 11 minutes a day. I think we should be aiming for that with our walking.

A brisk walk of 11 minutes every day could prevent one in 10 premature deaths worldwide, according to the largest ever study of its kind. Accumulating 75 minutes a week of moderate-intensity activity lowered the risk of early death by 23 per cent, researchers found. It was also enough to reduce the risk of cardiovascular disease by 17 per cent, and the risk of cancer by 7 per cent. This is such a good starting position – if you find that 11 minutes is manageable, then you could try stepping it up.

For more information see the section '11 minutes to change your life' starting on page 40.

Walk 3 minutes every half-hour

Indoor Step Snack

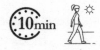

A great way to get your steps in while indoors.

This snack will get your heart pumping in just 10 minutes.

Method

Just crank up your music and set a timer; go as fast or as slow as you want. Vary the pace and intensity, based on your energy.

1. **Heel kicks**: Walk, jog or run on the spot, flicking your heels up to your bum.

2. **Walk, jog or run on the spot**: Standing, or you can even try simply marching on the spot while sitting on the sofa, going at your own pace.

3. **Step touch**: Step from side to side while reaching across with the opposite arm.

4. **Shuffle step or forward leaps**: Jump and land on both feet in a squat; shuffle-step back.

5. **Leg curls**: Step sideways, keeping low (squatting) and curl your heel to your bum.

6. **Boxing shuffles**: Walk, jog or run on the spot while punching your arms out – tins or light dumbbells are perfect for this.

7. **Step forwards and back**: Simply take a few steps forward and back, fast or slow, to the beat.

8. **High knees**: Lift your alternate knees towards your navel and tense your lower abs – move fast or slow, for low or high impact.

9. **Wide to narrow squat steps**: Step out to a wide squat; step feet in to a narrow squat. Keep going!

10. **Star jumps**: Step one or both feet in and out, with arms meeting to clap above your head – with or without jumping.

Benefits

- Great cardio for the heart, lungs and respiratory system
- Boosts mood
- Releases endorphins and Feels Good!

Top tips

- Put your favourite music playlist on – music is one of the best movement motivators. Pump it up and add in some dance snacks.
- Move and swing the arms as you do the moves, to work more of your body.

Back Snack

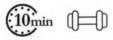

Strengthen your back to reduce back and neck pain, improve your posture, gain definition and future-proof your body. Trust me, this works!

I began incorporating back snacks into my weekly training programme when I started my perimenopause, from the age of forty, and I no longer suffer from the chronic back pain I endured in my twenties and thirties.

Equipment

- Some tin cans, plastic bottles or weights
- A long resistance band or a pair of old tights

Method

10 exercises in 10 minutes, focused on building a strong, sexy pain-free back.

Do as many reps as you can in one minute of each of the moves. The last few reps should be harder, almost to the point of failure, while maintaining good form (keeping your back straight, core engaged and muscles strong).

Progress from light weights to heavier weights gradually, over time, as your strength increases. Once you can't go heavier, play around with the tempo. The slower you go, the more time under tension for the muscles, so tempo is a great way to progress and get stronger. You could also shorten your rest periods or add more reps.

1. **Superwoman**: Lie on the floor facedown, with your legs straight and arms extended in front. Keeping your head neutral and looking down, lift your arms and legs a few inches off the floor. Engage your glutes, your core, and lift your belly button off the floor to contract your abs. Like you're a Superwoman flying in the air. Hold for a few seconds, then lower and repeat.

2. **Bird dog**: Start on your hands and knees with the hands under the shoulders and the knees under the hips. Extend one leg and the opposite arm at the same time. Pause for a few seconds, return to the starting position, and switch sides.

3. **Banded lateral pull-down**: Hold the resistance band with both hands; extend one arm up and keep it fixed straight by your ear; bend the elbow of the other arm down and out to the side while squeezing the muscles in your back and shoulder blades. Repeat this on the other side.

4. **Single arm row**: Using an elevated surface, keep your supporting arm straight. Bring the elbow of the arm performing the row close to the side of your body.

5. **Bent-over row**: It's like the RDL position (see page 175). Keep your elbows close to the side of your body as you row, pulling the dumbbells up towards the sides of your chest as you exhale. Lower the weights in a slow, controlled manner back to the starting position as you inhale.

6. **Reverse fly**: Lean forward in the RDL position (see page 175), letting your arms hang down next to your calves, with your elbows slightly bent. Slowly raise the weights until your elbows are level with your shoulders. Then slowly lower the weights to the starting position.

7. **Upright row**: Back straight, head held high, core tight; lead with your elbows as they draw up and out, into a hanger position at the top, with elbows at shoulder height; squeeze your back muscles and then lower your arms to the starting position.

8. **Renegade row**: From a high plank position, row the weight into the side of your body, drawing the elbows inwards and upwards, and not tilting/tipping your back or pelvis.

9. **Lateral raises**: Lift and lower your straight arms to the side, at shoulder height, and then down – tin cans are perfect for these. Repeat.

10. **Resistance band pull apart**: Really squeeze your shoulder blades together as the straight arms hold your resistance band or tights; pull open wide and come back, squeezing the shoulder blades together, in fast movements.

Benefits

- Improves stability
- Relieves lower back pain
- Strengthens your core, hips and back muscles
- Helps promote proper posture
- Increases the range of motion
- Supports healthy ageing

Next steps

- Before you do this snack, warm up, prime and prep with the Upper Body Mobility Snack on page 163.
- Always stretch it out by ending with the 5 minutes Post-Workout Upper Body Stretch Snack on page 177, the Feel Good Finish Snack on page 82 or the 10 minute End of Day Stretch Snack on page 92, if you have more time.

Top tips

- Keep your back fixed straight, with your spine long and strong, and always engage your core (draw your belly button towards your spine).
- Remember to breathe throughout, using exhales during the harder part of the move as you lift the weights.

Squat Snack

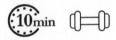

As the 'king' of lower body moves, it deserves its own snack, and you deserve it too – to build strong, powerful legs, glutes and core.

Compound movements like squats generate a high calorie burn. With all these variations you'll never get bored of squatting (and nor will your muscles) – once you master the basic squat, this will keep things interesting and help with motivation.

Equipment

- Some tins, plastic bottles or weights
- A small looped resistance band or a pair of old tights
- A weighted rucksack (filled with naughty fizzy drink cans)
- A chair/bed/sofa to give the pistol squats a go

Method

How to squat: Begin with just your bodyweight, then add in some resistance bands or light weights and increase them gradually over time. Always make sure your knees go out in line with your toes (not inwards), keeping your back straight and upright, core tight (suck in your belly button towards your spine) and bodyweight in your heels. Remember to breathe throughout, using exhales during the harder part of the move as you're coming back up to standing position, and squeeze your glutes at the top too.

Using tempo is a great way to challenge yourself and progress also. By slowing each move (both ways – down and up) the muscles are under tension for longer. For a gentle eccentric snack, slowly lower yourself, taking 3–5 seconds to do so, then come slowly back up again. Do this at least 10 times. If you are a squat queen, you could try doing this on one leg, which will also improve your balance.

You can play around with time too. Start with doing each move for 30 seconds, with 30 seconds rest in between. Then increase the work period to, say, 40 seconds, with 20 seconds rest in between. Then progress as you gain strength to doing each move for 1 minute, with no rest in between. Hardcore!

1. **Squat walk**: Place the resistance band, if using one, above your knees. Stand, chest proud, head and feet facing forward, abs braced, knees slightly bent. Point your feet forward, slightly wider than a hip distance apart. Maintain tension in the band or keep the squat width. Lower into a squat, forcing your knees out (against the band). Take steps sideways, leading with your knees, for as much space as you can.

2. **Normal squat**: Standing with feet just over a shoulder width apart, visualize sitting down on an imaginary seat, keeping your knees out in line with your toes, with your weight in your heels. Come back up to standing, squeezing your glutes at the top. (As you go down

and up, check you can see your toes so your knees are staying back.)

3. **Squat with side leg raise**: Squat down; as you come up to standing, lift one leg out straight to the side; then squat and repeat on the other side.

4. **Narrow squat**: Squat with a narrower stance, feet closer together, to target the quads at the front of the thighs.

5. **Sumo squat**: Like the squats above, but your feet are in a much wider stance; you should feel these in your inner and outer thighs and glutes as you go down and up.

6. **Single-leg pistol squats**: A single-leg squat with a box or chair half a step behind you. The goal is to sit down slowly and push yourself up, keeping one leg in the air the whole time.

7. **Squat pulses**: Squat with small pulses up and down at the bottom quarter of the squat.

8. **Sumo squat pulses**: Lower your body into a wider squat position and do small pulses up and down.

9. **Wall sit**: Squat against a wall. Take a seat against a wall, keeping back straight; knees at 90 degrees to the floor; core muscles engaged. Hold for as long as you can!

10. **Squat jumps**: Stand with your feet a shoulder width apart and the knees pointing outward in the same direction as your toes. Bend your knees, pressing your hips back as if you were going to sit back on a chair. Pushing through the heels, jump straight up. Land lightly, with your knees slightly bent, and go back into the squat position. Keep repeating, and when tired just go into normal, fast squats.

Benefits

- Strengthens your core and decreases belly fat
- Makes everyday movements like turning, bending and even standing easier
- Improves your balance
- Eases lower back pain
- Improves posture
- Reduces the risk of injury by strengthening your tendons, ligaments and bones
- Boosts athletic performance and strength
- Can be done anywhere
- Great for the brain (see the squats in the Superbrain Snack on page 287 for a variation)

Next steps

- Go for a Feel Good Walk Snack on page 207 and do this snack in the park (or even in the driveway). Alternatively, if you want to do it indoors, begin with the 5 minutes Lower Body Mobility Snack on page 169 to warm up the muscles.
- Make sure you stretch it out afterwards by doing the 5 minutes Post-Workout Lower Body Stretch Snack on page 180, or even the Standing Stretch Snack on page 147 too.
- Bonus 3 minute challenge: search for the song 'Bring Sally Up/Down' on YouTube or your music provider, and squat along to it!
- Bonus wall sit challenge: aim to build up to 2 minutes, as this isometric exercise is effective in lowering blood pressure.

Top tips

- You can practise your squats in front of a chair, so you touch it as you go down and to practise your technique.
- If you can't manage this whole squat snack, just think about adding in 10 squats a few times during your day. Then spice it up later with some of these variations. I have a friend who has embraced my squat snack advice and has tied it on to every time she goes to the toilet – that's her cue to do 10 squats. Genius, as it's piggybacking and anchored on to a habit. She can do them anywhere, and nobody even knows she's doing them!

Squat for longevity and a healthy brain

If you can do nothing else in regards to strength training, do Squat Snacks (see page 221)! Squats strengthen your lower body muscles, which are some of your largest and most powerful muscles – hence so important to work!

The ability to get in and out of a chair is a really good indicator of your future health. Squats simulate probably the most common movement pattern we do every day. When you have to go to the washroom, that's a squat. When you get in the car, that's a squat. Every time you sit down or stand up, that's a squat. If you don't do them well, it affects the way you live. Research shows a link between strong leg muscles and longevity. One study that followed healthy adults aged seventy and older for more than six years found that those who had greater quadriceps strength had a lower risk of early death.

According to Dr Damian Bailey, Director of the Neuro-vascular Research Laboratory at the University of South Wales, squats are the best exercise to boost your brain health. Simple squats – where you go up (working against gravity) and where you go down (working with gravity) – increase and decrease the blood flow to your brain. While you squat, the blood flow to the hippocampus increases, which is the region of the brain principally responsible for learning and memory faculties (which naturally begin to decrease as we age).

Squats also stimulate the release of the brain fertilizer BDNF, which literally leads to the growth of new brain cells and connections. The research shows that just 3 to 5 minutes of squats, 3 times a week, can be better for your brain than

30 minutes of steady-state exercise, such as a run or a walk, which takes much longer and more of your time.

To further push and challenge your brain you could listen to a podcast, or read or try a crossword while doing your squats. Or stay engaged and part of a Zoom meeting, but just switch your camera off – the perfect time to do squats when you are working! If you want to mix things up, press-ups also give the up–down movement of squats, working against gravity too.

The best thing is that you can do some really easy little exercises and snacks that don't really feel like you're exercising at all – and it won't get you sweaty, so you can squat anywhere!

Lower Body Strength and Cardio Snack

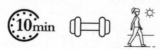

A special mix of cardio and strength to challenge you.

Warning: this may be tough and one you want to build up to as you get fitter and stronger. For the HIIT moves you can do them low impact without the jumps too.

Equipment

All you need are some tin cans, plastic bottles (or weights in the future).

Method

You can challenge yourself with time.

Start with doing each move for 30 seconds, with 30 seconds rest in between. Then increase the work period to, say, 40 seconds, with 20 seconds rest in between. Then progress as you gain strength to doing each move for 1 minute, with no rest in between. Hardcore!

Refer to the Lower Body Strength Snack on page 114 and the cardio HIIT Snack on page 97 for specific exercise tips.

1. **Froggers**: Stand with your feet spread wider than shoulder width apart. Bend at the knees; sink into a low squat and place your palms in prayer position, pushing your knees out with your elbows. To progress you can place your palms on the ground slightly in front of you and try to straighten your legs out, then bring them back to a low squat/frog position (often called the yogi squat).

2. **High knees**: Lift your alternate knees towards your navel and tense your lower abs – move fast or slow, for low or high impact.

3. **Squats**: Visualize sitting back on an imaginary seat, keeping your knees out in line with your toes, and then squeezing your glutes as you come back up.

4. **Sprint or march**: On the spot.

5. **Reverse lunges**: From a standing position, take a long stride back so the front knee doesn't go over the front foot; try to bend both knees at a 90 degree angle; keep your body straight as you lower (not leaning forwards); lift your back heel up and place your weight in the heel of front foot. Step back in and repeat on alternate sides.

6. **Squats in and out**: Jump or step from wide to narrow.

7. **Side lunges**: Take a long step out to the side, keeping feet parallel; bend and sink into the leg you stepped out with, while keeping the other leg straight. Then return back to standing and alternate sides.

8. **Curtsy lunges**: Putting your weight into your front foot, step back and around with your other foot – almost as if you're curtsying. Ensure that your chest stays proud. Stop lunging when your right thigh is parallel to the ground.

Begin to straighten your front leg, pushing up through your heel, and returning your back foot to the starting position.

9. **Glute bridges (single or doubles)**: Lying on your back, knees bent, a hip width apart; imprint your back into the ground; exhale as you peel back off the mat and squeeze your glutes tight at the top of the move; lift hips as high as you can; then inhale as you lower. Do single leg for a harder option.

10. **Mountain climbers**: From a high plank position, alternate bringing one knee in to your chest, then back out again.

Benefits

- Increased calorie burn
- Improved cardiovascular health
- Increased muscle mass
- Increased strength and power
- Better bone density
- Increased endurance
- Improved mental health

Next steps

- Begin with the 5 minutes Lower Body Mobility Snack on page 169 to prep the muscles.
- Make sure you stretch it out by doing the 5 minutes Post-Workout Lower Body Stretch Snack on page 180 at the end, and even the Standing Stretch Snack on page 147 too.

Top tips

- Do the moves with just your bodyweight, build up your strength slowly, then incorporate weights.
- Remember to breathe throughout; don't hold your breath or you may experience the 'valsalva' effect when people say they feel sick or dizzy as they don't breathe enough oxygen in when exercising.
- Music may be a great idea to get you through this snack!

Cardio, Core and Upper Body Strength Snack

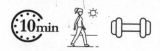

A combination of cardio, core and upper body strength moves to really challenge you. It's full body and done in just 10 minutes if you commit to it!

A challenging combination of moves which will work your core, get you out of breath and then test your fitness by moving straight into a strength exercise. You could do this once or twice a week if you're hardcore!

Equipment

All you need are some weights – tin cans, plastic bottles or dumbbells.

Method

Start with just your bodyweight, then add in some weights over time. You can do the HIIT moves low impact, without the jumps, as a modification. Keep your back straight and upright, core tight (suck in your belly button towards your spine) and remember to breathe throughout, don't hold your breath.

10 moves in 10 minutes – do as much as you can!

Maybe start with doing each move for 30 seconds, with 30 seconds rest in between.

Then increase the work period to, say, 40 seconds, with 20 seconds rest in between.

Then progress as you gain strength by doing each move for 1 minute, with no rest in between. Tough!

1. **Press-ups**: Keep your back straight, core tight; bring your chest between your hands and bend your arms at 90 degrees; progress with depth, tempo and level – you can start at a wall and then an incline surface, progressing to the floor, in a box, three-quarters or full plank position.

2. **Cross-body climbers**: From a plank position, alternate bringing one knee to your opposite elbow, then back out again.

3. **Arnold press**: Hold the weights right in front of your shoulders at collarbone height with your hands facing you, unlike a regular shoulder press. As you press the weights up, rotate your hands to face away from you. Drive the weights upwards until your elbows are fully extended; then control the weights back to the starting position.

4. **High knees with ropes**: Lift one knee at a time up towards your chest while imagining pulling a rope with alternate arms.

5. **Lateral and front raises**: Lift straight arms to the front (to shoulder height) then down; then lift to your side (to shoulder height) and down. Repeat.

6. **Boxing**: Punch all your worries away while walking, jogging or sprinting on the spot. Vary punches to the front, upwards and sideways.

7. **Low to high plank**: Start in a low plank with forearms on the floor; in a controlled motion, push up with one arm at a time into a high plank with hands on the floor. Check that your shoulders are stacked over your elbows/hands and that your body is in one straight line. Proceed back down, lowering one forearm to the floor at a time. Repeat and keep alternating sides.

8. **Burpees**: Stand with your feet a shoulder width apart. Bend at your hips and knees to lower yourself into a squatting position. Place your hands on the floor in front of you. Step or jump your feet back so that you are in a high plank position. Step or jump your feet back towards your hands and jump or straighten up to standing.

9. **Bent-over row**: It's like the RDL position (see page 175). Keep your elbows close to the side of your body as you row, pulling the dumbbells up towards the sides of your chest as you exhale. Lower the weights in a slow, controlled manner back to the starting position as you inhale.

10. **Star jumps**: Step one or both legs in and out, with arms meeting to clap above your head – with or without jumping.

Benefits

- Gets the heart pumping
- Boosts your bone health

- Strengthens upper body muscles
- Keeps you motivated

Next steps

- Begin with the 5 minutes Upper Body Mobility Snack on page 163 and/or the Desk/Sofa Snack on page 157 to warm up the muscles.
- Make sure you stretch it out by doing the 5 minutes Post-Workout Upper Body Stretch Snack on page 177 at the end. And the long End of Day Stretch Snack on page 92 may be needed.

Top tips

- You could take this snack outdoors on your Feel Good Walk Snack on page 207 – the fresh air may help keep you cool.
- Music may be a great idea to get you through this snack.

Legs, Bums and Tums Snack

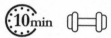

Back to the 1990s with this combo snack. A golden oldie name – and isn't it still what women want?

I promise you this snack won't disappoint. This is a good one!

Equipment

- Some optional weights
- A looped resistance band
- A mat or a rug

Method

Start with just your bodyweight or a resistance band. Then add in some weights, if you want.

10 moves in 10 minutes. LBT focuses on your lower body, so you'll work on a combination of exercises targeting your legs, stomach and glutes.

1. **Curtsy lunges**: Putting your weight into your front foot, step back and around with your other foot – almost as if you're curtsying. Back straight, chest proud. Stop

lunging when your right thigh is parallel to the ground. Begin to straighten your front leg, pushing up through your heel, and returning your back foot to the starting position.

Or reverse lunges: From a standing position, take a long step backwards with one foot (with heel off the ground). Bend your front knee until it's at a 90 degree angle, and lower your back knee towards the ground until it is also bent at a right angle. Then push back up and return to the starting position. Repeat on alternate sides.

2. **Standing cross-body crunches**: Standing straight, bring your hands behind your head, elbows pointing out to the sides. Twist your body, bringing your elbow down and across while raising the opposite knee to meet it. Return to the starting position and keep alternating sides.

3. **Glute bridges**: Lying on your back, knees bent, a hip width apart, imprint your back into the ground; peel your back off the mat; lift your hips as high as you can and squeeze your glutes tight at the top of the move.

4. **Bicycles**: Hold your head gently with your hands, elbows out. Lift your feet from the floor to a bicycle pedal motion, bringing one knee up towards your armpit while straightening the other leg and also rotating your torso. Twist so you can touch your elbow to the opposite knee as it comes up. Keep alternating sides.

5. **Donkey kicks**: On all fours, knees a hip width apart, hands under your shoulders, neck and spine neutral. Bracing your core, begin to lift your right leg, knee staying bent, foot staying flat, and hinging at the hip.

Use your glute to press your foot directly towards the ceiling, and squeeze at the top. Ensure your pelvis and hips stay parallel, pointing towards the ground. Return to the starting position. 30 seconds on each side. Try with a resistance band tied around your thigh or ankles.

6. **Romanian Deadlifts (RDLs)**: Begin by standing with your feet a hip width apart and knees slightly bent. Hold one weight in each hand, and place them in front of your hips, with palms facing thighs. Keeping your spine straight in a neutral position and squeezing your shoulder blades, core tight, start sending your hips back. (You want to feel this in the back of your legs, at the top, as the hips hinge and travel back – practise in front of a wall, imagining closing a car door with your bottom.) Keeping the weights close to your body, lower them down so they are in front of your shins. Maintain a neutral spine and drive through your heels to fully extend hips and knees as you come back up to standing, squeezing your glutes at the top.

7. **Clams**: Lie on your side, legs together and knees bent. With your feet together, slowly raise your right knee. Activate your side abs and squeeze your glutes. Hold for a few seconds, then lower back to the starting position. Both sides for 30 seconds. As you get stronger, place a resistance band around the thighs to make the move harder.

8. **Side planks**: Lie on one side, legs extended and stacked from hip to feet. The elbow of your arm is directly under your shoulder. Lift your hips and knees from the mat while exhaling and engaging your core tight. Your torso

is straight in line, with no sagging or bending. Hold the position for up to 30 seconds on both sides.

9. **Sumo squats**: Like normal squats, but your feet are in a much wider stance and you should feel the stretch in your inner and outer thighs and glutes as you go down and up. Add in pulses by squatting down, pushing a quarter of the way back up, and pulse up and down from there.

10. **Spider-Man plank**: Start in low/forearm plank position. Pull your right knee towards the outside of your right elbow and then push it back to return to a plank position. Alternate sides. If this is too hard, just hold a low plank for as long as possible.

Benefits

- Targets many of the largest muscles in your body
- Builds strength and muscle mass
- Tones your legs, glutes and abs
- Helps you get fitter
- Improves muscle tone
- Helps maintain good balance and stability
- Aids mobility and flexibility
- Boosts mood and energy too

Next steps

- Begin with the 5 minutes Lower Body Mobility Snack on page 169 and/or the Fitness Salutation Snack on page 124 to warm up the muscles.
- If you have time, add on a 1 minute or 5 minute HIIT Snack on page 97.

Top tips

- Keep your core tight throughout (suck in your belly button towards your spine).
- Stretch well with the 5 minutes Post-Workout Lower Body Stretch Snack on page 180 at the end, or even the 5 minutes Seated Stretch Snack on page 192 if you're tired.
- Set up a playlist of motivating tunes!

Bed
Stretch Snack

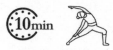

Ideal as a nightcap to aid restful sleep and stretch out the day, or lovely in the morning for those times when we find it hard to get out of bed, and to start the day with some self-care.

I recommend making this a habit every evening before you go to sleep. Many of these moves will help the parasympathetic nervous system to kick in, to calm the body and mind for rest, especially as you tie in your breath with each stretch.

Method

If you want to, set a timer for 10 minutes, or just listen to your body and spend as much time as you need on each move.

1. **Seated forward fold**: Sit with your legs straight in front of you. Inhale and reach with both arms towards the ceiling, arms parallel to your ears. As you exhale, keep on reaching forward, and bend forward, reaching with your hands towards your toes or as far as you can go. Hold, relax and breathe.

2. **Seated feel-good hug**: See the Feel Good Hug Snack on page 80. This is like a seated cat/cow with a lovely self-hug.

3. **Seated butterfly**: Sit with the soles of your feet pressing into each other. Elongate and straighten your spine, tucking your chin in towards your chest. Fall heavy towards your soles and relax or sink a bit more deeply into the stretch with your breath. To deepen the intensity, move your feet closer in towards your hips.

4. **Seated spinal twist**: Sit cross-legged, bring left hand to your right knee and place the right hand's fingertips on the mat behind you. Inhale, sit up tall and lengthen your spine. Exhale, twist from the base of your spine to the right. Repeat on the other side.

5. **Lying feel-good hug**: Lying with your knees bent, lift your knees towards your chest. Place your hands around both knees and draw them towards your chest. Hug in and release/massage your lower back, maybe rocking side to side or drawing circles with your knees.

6. **Glute stretch**: On your back with your knees bent, cross your left foot over your right quad. Lift your right leg off the floor. Grab on to the back of your right leg and gently pull it towards your chest. Hold for up to 30 seconds on each side.

7. **Lower back stretch**: Lying on your back, bring your arms out to the sides with the palms facing down in a T position. Bend the right knee and pull it to twist over to the left side of your body. Look at the right fingertips, keeping shoulders grounded. Repeat on the other side.

8. **Happy baby**: Lying flat on your back, bring your knees towards your chest, keeping them at a 90 degree angle. Reach forward and grab the inside or outside edges of your feet – whatever's most comfy. Spread your knees apart gently. Flex your ankles and gently rock from side to side (like a happy baby).

9. **Legs up headboard**: Lie down on your back and try to get your bum as close to the headboard or a wall as possible, extending your legs up, perpendicular to the floor. Open your arms to the sides, palms up. Flex your feet for an added hamstring stretch. If that's too uncomfortable, you can scoot away a bit so your legs are at an easier angle.

10. **Corpse pose**: Lie down fully and separate your legs. Bring your arms alongside but slightly separated from your body, palms up. Fully relax all your limbs and release any effort from holding them in position. Let your breathing occur naturally for ultimate relaxation.

Benefits

- Encourages a better night's sleep
- Improves blood flow
- Relieves muscle tension
- Calms the body and mind
- Releases any tightness
- Loosens the muscles
- Can reduce soreness from exercise

Next steps

- Stack on a breath snack (perhaps Mindful Minute 4–6 Breath Snack on page 283 or Mindful Minute 5.5 Breath Snack on page 273).
- Or select something from the menu of self-care snacks and nibbles on page 269.

Top tips

- Muscles stretch best when they are warm, so ideally create a bedtime ritual that involves heat, such as taking a warm bath or shower before (see the Heat Snack on page 341).
- Turn down the lights, perhaps light a candle and play some relaxing music – see my 'Top tips to help you feel good with sleep' on page 315.

Feel Good Mentally

I have heard of so many women going to their doctor through perimenopause and menopause and being prescribed antidepressants. Consistent exercise has been shown to be just as, if not more, effective as antidepressant medications for those with major depression. (However, please note that antidepressants may be needed – everyone's situation and treatment is case by case and should be assessed by a qualified medical professional.) Yet exercise is probably one of the most under-utilized forms of therapy for mental health. In fact, a large new meta-analysis of studies published in the *British Journal of Sports Medicine* found that essentially all forms of exercise produced significant mental health benefits. Shorter, high-intensity exercise programmes produced the greatest effect, in line with exercise snacking.

Preliminary evidence also suggests that physically active people have lower rates of anxiety and depression than sedentary people. According to the *Journal of Clinical Psychiatry*, exercise improves mental health by reducing anxiety, depression and negative mood. And it improves self-esteem and cognitive function. This is particularly useful during menopause when anxiety and low mood are common symptoms. It has also been found to help with building social connection, which is key to midlife and long-term health. For more on this, see the section on 'Social snacking' starting on page 325.

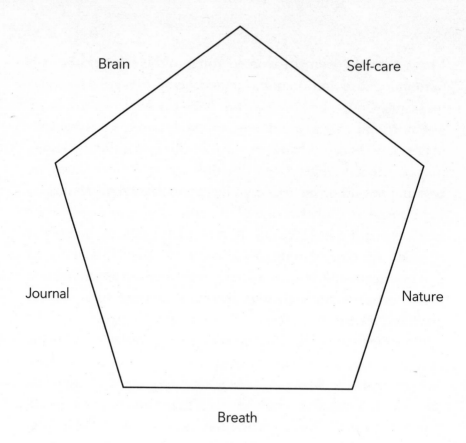

Brain

Self-care

Journal

Nature

Breath

The benefits of exercise for mental health

Working out will truly make you feel good. Benefits include:

- reduced stress levels
- increased energy levels
- reduced depression
- increased mood and well-being
- reduced anxiety
- increased self-esteem and confidence
- improved sleep
- increased brain power.

Besides the physical and psychological benefits of exercise, the rush of feel-good chemicals (endorphins) you'll get are an added bonus. This can be especially important for women going through menopause. Our bodies are experiencing a number of changes that may be uncomfortable and even painful. Exercise can help you through this phase of life and leave you feeling better than ever.

It's important to note that every woman experiences menopause differently, and not every woman feels her best during this time. And that's okay. But if you're feeling blue, you'll be happy to know that exercise can be the free pick-me-up you need to help you feel good about yourself. One study found that, over time, physical activity was associated with higher levels of self-worth and menopause-related quality of life.

Alongside our mental health, self-care is also an essential part of the journey to feeling good. I've dabbled in meditation and enjoyed yoga since my thirties but it's only since entering the peri-menopause that I've really started to prioritize my own self-care and have developed a consistent toolbox that I enjoy and use on a daily basis. I turned to self-care methods just to keep me sane and reduce anxiety, worries and calm myself down, as I was juggling so many different things, like all mothers out there.

There are several self-care methods in this book, but the main ones I now use regularly are breath work, stretch snacks, jour-naling, walking, and running a good old-fashioned bath. Let me explain some of these in more detail and then you can try them out and save them in your own Feel Good toolkit.

Give yourself permission to slow down

Brain

I understand that people exercise for different reasons. Many people stay fit to prevent serious health conditions like heart disease, obesity, diabetes and stroke; others work out primarily to lose weight. But I'm guessing only a few people exercise with the intent to boost and strengthen their brain. As well as the obvious benefits to your body, both internally and externally, exercise also benefits your brain.

Build the brain muscle

While we are focused on building muscles, we need to also build our brain. Studies have shown that a single exercise session can help enhance our cognitive abilities and improve mental focus better than a cup of coffee! Exercise can boost your brain power and also increase concentration levels by improving blood flow to the brain. Physical activity improves memory and learning. It also activates different parts of the brain and enables the release of the BDNF chemical as well as norepinephrine neurotransmitters; these increase alertness, concentration and energy. For more on this, see my work nibbles on page 336.

Never too late

As women, yes, we want to live longer but we want to do this happily and healthily, and the best way we can do this is to invest in our brain health from midlife, especially during peri-menopause and beyond. But if you are older and reading this, remember it's never too late! Exercise plays a huge role later on in life also, and there's so much you can do, so easily, whatever your age or ability.

A study in the *Journal of Alzheimer's Disease Reports* has found that brain connectivity and memory improves in older adults after walking. These results add to growing evidence that exercise slows cognitive impairment and may delay the onset of Alzheimer's disease. Regular walks strengthen connections in and between brain networks.

In another study, older adults with mild cognitive impairment who lifted weights 2 or 3 times a week improved cognitive function, as well as muscle tone. We know that, as women, we have a much higher risk of Alzheimer's disease – and especially after menopause – so this research is very promising and even more hopeful that exercise may be useful as a way to prevent onset and reduce our risk. (See Alzheimer's and dementia section on page 27.)

Brain boost tip

If you've got an important meeting, phone call or presentation, get an exercise snack in first to boost your brain power and performance. Tell your kids before they write a test or an exam, or go into an interview, or do anything that is cognitively demanding, they should get some exercise first as it will help them perform better.

Brain nibbles

- Simply get vertical. Just get out of the chair! Standing and adding in movement increases your blood flow, heart rate, changes your breathing, and encourages your brain to stay active.
- Do some star jumps. Packed with brain-boosting power, they'll pump blood to your brain.
- Snack on one of the 10 minutes cardio snacks. Studies show that just ten minutes can boost your brain power.
- Plank to clear your mind (for example, try the Core Snack on page 119 or the Full Body Strength Snack on page 172).
- Boost your brain power by going for a Feel Good Walk Snack (see page 207). A 2017 study found that the foot-to-ground impacts increase the amount of blood sent to the brain.
- Walking while you work can improve memory and attention (even after you've stopped walking).
- A breath snack can stimulate the vagus nerve to rewire your brain and reduce anxiety.
- Yoga helps boost memory and can also improve brain function and vitality (try my End of Day Stretch Snack on page 92).
- Gentle exercises like t'ai chi can influence brain activity and relieve stress. Numerous studies have concluded that it increases the size of the brain and enhances a person's brain power, memory and thinking and when done regularly can improve brain health, especially for elderly people.
- Lift weights! Systematic studies that have been conducted to assess the influence of weight-lifting exercises

show a highly positive impact on brain capacity, alertness, attention and memory. A combination of weight and resistance training exercises can increase brain power and brain health in people over the age of fifty.

- If you're new or haven't exercised in a while, don't fret. Those who are not as fit get the biggest brain benefits from exercise because their brains are not as used to cushioning the changes in blood flow. The more fluctuations in blood flow, the more good chemicals are released. Challenge yourself when you're ready. Combining exercise moves that require coordination, harder patterns and movement challenges can greatly improve memory and reasoning, particularly in people with mild cognitive impairment.

Journaling

When I was a teenager I used to write a diary and it was the best place for me to confess my secrets, struggles and fears without judgement or punishment. Let's hope it's still hidden away at my parents' house and no one has broken its special lock and key! Looking back, it felt really good to get all those thoughts and feelings out of my head and on to paper, especially during the hormonal years of puberty. The world seemed clearer as a result.

I restarted journaling, which is what the grown-ups call it, at the start of the pandemic. Not only has it helped me alleviate the anxiety during the lockdowns – which I can identify now as being one of my main perimenopausal symptoms – but it's also been a wonderful way for me to track, log and celebrate what have been the best experiences of my life on this new journey through midlife!

So if you stopped using a diary as you grew up, I'd urge you to restart. It will help you deal with any overwhelming feelings, especially if you struggle with stress, depression or anxiety, and it can help you gain control of your emotions and improve your mental health. It's also a great tool to track symptoms day to day (which I do in my perimenopause). It can help you recognize triggers and learn better ways to deal with them. It provides an opportunity for positive self-talk and allows you to simply write your worries away. It's also a great form of self-love, to celebrate your wins in your private journal.

The physical act of writing also engages the brain and activates the prefrontal cortex (which regulates our response to stressful situations).

Gratitude

Gratitude is the experience of counting your blessings and being thankful for what you have. I often call it vitamin G! During those hard times in life, especially in midlife and beyond, when we can experience emotions like overwhelm, grief, pain and anxiety, it can be hard to see the good things in life. But I think that during these challenging times, it's even more important to try and adopt an attitude of gratitude. This will help you to recognize when things are going right in your life instead of focusing on the negative.

Try some of the snacks in this book or even, every night, write down anything that made you say 'Yay!' during the day.

Breath

Breath snacks are perfect for those times when you are feeling anxious or stressed and need to reset your nervous system. By focusing on your breath, you are allowing the parasympathetic nervous system to kick in and help the body to rest, recover and digest. This is the opposite of the fight-or-flight response when in stressful situations. It's literally rewiring, resetting and recalibrating the nervous system.

You can work with your breath to bring back balance into your own ecosystem. It's so powerful. It will benefit your:

- immune system
- digestive system
- endocrine and reproductive system
- creativity
- performance
- energy levels
- sleep patterns.

Visualize yourself inhaling new energy, and then exhaling, getting rid of the old. Inhale positivity, exhale negativity.

According to the Mayo Clinic, there's sufficient evidence that intentional deep breathing can actually calm and regulate the autonomic nervous system (ANS) which regulates involuntary body functions such as temperature. It can lower blood pressure and provide an almost immediate sense of calm.

The slow holding of breath allows CO_2 to build up in the blood. This enhances the cardio-inhibitory response of the

When we breathe we reset ourselves

vagus nerve when you exhale and stimulates your parasympathetic system, hence producing a calm and relaxed feeling in the mind and body.

Did you know that a person has roughly 50,000 thoughts a day? This technique will declutter the mind and help the swarm of nagging thoughts leave your head. Give your mind a break – just a few minutes will be beneficial.

My own breath work practice has helped me immensely over the last few years since the pandemic, which is when I really started using this technique. Anytime I've felt overwhelmed or anxious, I've turned to my breath. It's been such a saviour during my perimenopause journey too.

The fact that you can do breath work anywhere, without any fancy equipment, at any time of day, makes it so easy. I have practised this exercise before going on TV or radio, doing public speaking or going live on social media – when the adrenaline is rushing around – to help me refocus and gain a sense of calm, and ease the nerves of course. I simply close my eyes and take a few deep breaths before I start.

My youngest son has seen me do deep breathing and long, loud exhales behind the steering wheel. At first, he thought I was very strange, but then I asked him to give it a go with me. It's now become normal on days when we are running late. Or when he has a test or an exam, we've started using it as a tool for him too. The car is sometimes the best place to do it as we are alone, and it's our quality time together without distractions.

As I am of the Jain religion, I was fascinated to read in James Nestor's book *Breath: The New Science of a Lost Art* that when Buddhist monks chant their most popular mantra, *om mani padme hum*, each spoken phrase lasts six seconds, with six seconds to inhale before the chant starts again. The traditional chant of *om*, the 'sacred sound of the universe', used in Jainism and other traditions, takes six seconds to sing, with a pause of about six seconds to inhale. He writes:

> In 2001, researchers at the University of Pavia in Italy gathered two dozen subjects, covered them with sensors to measure blood flow, heart rate, and nervous system feedback, then had them recite a Buddhist mantra as well as the original Latin version of the rosary, the Catholic prayer cycle of the Ave Maria, which is repeated half by a priest and half by the congregation. They were stunned to find the average number of breaths for each cycle was 'almost exactly' identical, just a bit quicker than the pace of the Hindu, Taoist, and Native American prayers: 5.5 breaths a minute . . .
>
> Whenever they followed this slow breathing pattern, blood flow to the brain increased, and the systems in the body entered a state of coherence where the functions of heart, circulation, and nervous system are coordinated to peak efficiency. The moment the subjects returned to spontaneous breathing or talking, their hearts would beat a little more erratically, and the integration of these systems would slowly fall apart. A few more slow and relaxed breaths, and it would return again . . .
>
> This resonant breathing offered the same benefits as meditation for people who didn't want to meditate. Or yoga for people who didn't like to get off the couch. It offered the healing touch of prayer for people who weren't religious.

I love that he talks about 'breath as prayer'. See my Mindful Minute 5.5 Breath Snack on page 273.

Mindful minute

I'm going to introduce you to a 'mindful minute'. All I'm asking for is 1 minute to start: that's all you need for one of my breath snacks, to start practising some of the techniques I've been sharing in my free Feel Good sessions. Pause and Practise! Give yourself permission to slow down. Use it as a secret tool at any time, wherever you are. It only takes 1 minute to clear the blood-stream of adrenaline and cortisol – proof that, sometimes, a minute is all you need.

Wherever you are, just sit back, find some stillness, close your eyes, focus on your breath, and count with me. Then move on to some of my other breath snacks to add to your Feel Good mind toolkit.

Nature

The research is clear: regular walking can help women cope with some of the symptoms of menopause. I have always encouraged people to go on 'walk snacks', but ideally outside in nature. It's my therapy, and it's so good for us to be outside and in some greenery. I always feel the incredible mental health benefits, even from just a short bout of being outside in the fresh air. Walking is my therapy. I find the mental health benefits of walking outdoors in nature so incredible and I've had many of my most creative brainwaves and work ideas on my Feel Good walks. I walk all year round, rain or shine. I just wrap up well and head out into the elements. Even if it's only for 5 minutes, I feel better for it!

Whether you go for a walk, run, cycle, outdoor swim or simply take your workout/snack outside, ideally expose yourself to some time outdoors. Nature really is a healer.

I remember how therapeutic my walks were during the Covid lockdowns and through those years of undiagnosed perimenopausal symptoms when I was at the start of my virtual workouts and stepping out on a new path. They were like a lifeline, so that's when I decided to research the power of nature further.

Research has found that time spent in green outdoor spaces can lower blood pressure and cortisol levels and is associated with better brain and body health. Over 100 studies have shown that being in nature, living near nature, or even viewing nature in paintings and videos, can have a positive impact on our brain, body, feelings, thought processes and social interactions. In particular, viewing nature seems to be inherently rewarding, producing a cascade of positive emotions and calming our nervous system. These, in turn, help us to cultivate greater openness, creativity, connection, generosity and resilience.

Fractals

A 'fractal' is a pattern that the laws of nature repeat at different scales. Exact fractals are ordered in such a way that the same basic pattern repeats exactly at every scale, like the growth spiral of a plant, for example. In a forest, you can find hundreds of fractals, if you look for them – from seeds and pine cones to the similar replication of trees and ferns.

Studies show that exposure to fractal patterns in nature reduces stress levels by up to 60 per cent. Give it a go on your Feel Good Walk Snacks (see page 207)! See how fractals can bring some calm and relaxation to your day.

Nature for the win!

The majority of middle-aged women report being dissatisfied with their bodies, with as few as 12 per cent of women being satisfied with the way they look. Poor body image in menopause poses additional risks to mental health; middle-aged women who report being dissatisfied with their bodies experience depression nearly twice as much as women who are satisfied with their bodies. Studies on the effects of outdoor exercise on body image and self-esteem in postmenopausal women showed that those who participated in outdoor exercise had higher self-esteem, better mood and greater body satisfaction than those who did not.

There are such incredible benefits for menopausal women in

getting outdoors and immersing themselves in nature, including the benefits it has on stress, sleep and mental health. In other words, science suggests we may seek out nature not only for our physical survival but also because it's good for our mental, social and personal well-being.

Self-care

What is self-care?

To me self-care is ring-fencing time every day to restore my physical, mental, emotional, spiritual and hormonal balance. It doesn't need to be long; even a 1 minute, 3 minutes or 5 minutes self-care snack is often enough for me to put myself first and does the job in terms of caring for and prioritizing myself. Self-care is a way to reclaim your power, especially in this chaotic fast-paced world. Making time for self-care is important for building resilience to help you cope with those stressors in life that are outside your control. When I invest in myself this way, it really increases my happiness, focus, stability, joy, peace and self-love. I feel more fulfilled, less anxious, no longer torn in multiple directions, as I've given myself that time and space to recalibrate my body and mind.

Mums – well, women in general – tend to put their own needs on the back burner, but even just a few minutes of me-time will help you reboot. One study found that choosing to be alone for just 15 minutes could lead to more relaxation and less stress. Remember, you can even snack your way up in smaller time increments. Self-care is about recognizing your needs and then fulfilling them. And as with everything in this book, there is no cost associated!

Let me give you a personal example. I had been worrying about the endless list of things to do and was experiencing feelings of overwhelm when writing this chapter of the book. I had got frustrated with a long school run in awful traffic, and was feeling more and more stressed. So I decided to go for a

10 minute walk round the block as soon as I got home (not even enter the front door, so I didn't get pulled into doing the house-work). A nice brisk walk with my pup Bailey worked like magic! It cleared my mind and de-stressed me. Just looking up at the sky and feeling the natural daylight energized me. I came back to my desk, calm and alert, and set my pomodoro timer and wrote this section for a productive 25 minutes. I've tried and tested this same method with lots of the exercise snacks in this book. Just a little bit of movement before you start your work, or if you face something difficult, always helps. Give it a go, it's one of my favourite hacks.

Self-care isn't selfish

Many people, unfortunately, see self-care as a luxury rather than a priority, and as a result are often left feeling tired, overwhelmed and ill equipped to handle life's inevitable challenges. It's time to change the narrative. Self-care isn't selfish, especially not for us women!

I'm really passionate about this issue, being South Asian, where women tend to have large family responsibilities and the culture is all about looking after others. So, for example, going to the gym or working out can be seen as selfish. I understand this, as I used to live in an extended family, with nine people including my in-laws, and although they would support me, it can be tricky for more traditional families, where the importance of exercise may not be fully understood. Women may feel that investing in self-care takes away time that should be spent in the home, or with the family, or working or caring for others. I argue that if you take the time out to do exercise, or any form of self-care, and something to support your own physical and mental health, then everyone around you will benefit from it too. You'll be healthier, stronger and in a better mood, so your relationships will benefit. You will be mentally and physically fitter too.

Look after yourself, so you can look after those around you better too. Self-care is one of the most important things we can advocate for ourselves.

How to practise self-care

I know it can seem difficult to carve out time for self-care but it's so important to dedicate a few minutes every day to looking after yourself. Just a little bit every day will add up and make a big difference in the long run. There are so many exercises in this book that I would classify as self-care, as they are all investing in your health and give you that important me-time. Turn to the mood menus at the back of the book, starting on page 365, to see what you fancy, based on how you're feeling.

Try out some activities, it's not a one-size-fits-all strategy. Highlight the snacks, or put a sticky note on the page, or jot down the page numbers in your journal, so you find out which ones help you. Find your own favourites – it's very personal. You want to have a feeling of rejuvenation after the activity; it should be recharging your battery, rather than depleting it. Remember, at first, it may not come easy to you! We hear so many people talking about the 'self-care trend' these days, but everyone is different. That's why microdosing my snacks and exposing yourself to a little at a time is a good way to introduce new habits, and it should start feeling good eventually. Be wary about the flipside and feeling that self-care is becoming a chore – or feeling slightly self-punishing – we definitely don't want that!

I want you to find methods that feel like a real, well-deserved treat. If you view Sundays, like I do, as Self-care Sundays (something I've been sharing on social media for years), that's a great way for you to schedule some self-care. Look forward to it, as a weekly ritual and a chance to recharge.

Make time to do things you love

I'm one of those people who usually prefer to move in order to feel better, but over the years I have become so happy in my own company and have grown to love stillness too. I try to listen to my body, my mood, my hormones, and pick something that feels right at the time. It's like a little gift to myself, even if it's only a few minutes.

The mindful walks I do are like radical self-care. These walks are without distractions or devices. The connection to nature, the surroundings and my senses is so powerful. It gives me space to solve issues; to create, generate and produce new ideas; to invigorate and be at one with myself. I can hear and listen to my body and turn off all the external noise. I may take the same route and path, so the familiarity allows me to be free and creative, and I don't have to think or worry about the direction. Add this technique into your Feel Good Walk Snack on page 207.

Self-care is important, and you deserve to make it a priority.

Self-care nibbles

Here's a menu of other self-care ideas and activities you can try.

- **Stillness:** Just be still and do nothing!
- **Solitude Snack:** Me-time (or time alone) gives you space to take the pressure off, recharge, get to know yourself and improve your mental health.

- **Hair oiling and scalp massage**: The practice of pouring oil on to the hair and massaging it into the scalp.
- **Tapping Snack**: Tapping the 12 meridian points of the body.
- **Face massage/rolling**: This can improve your mood, reduce anxiety, and help enhance the look of your skin.
- **Make-up Snack**: Take time to enjoy getting dolled up.
- **Skincare Snack**: Apply your skincare routine and massage it in, enjoying each step.
- **Face Mask Snack**: Time out to rest and relax while putting on your favourite face mask.
- **Singing/Dancing Snack**: A good old sing-song and boogie to your favourite track.
- **Music Snack**: Listen to a song you love.
- **Love letter to yourself**: 'Dear Me, I love how you . . . I'm proud of you for . . . I know you feel loved when . . .'
- **Meditation**: There are so many forms of meditation to focus and clear your mind and be still.
- **Coffee/tea ritual**: Just the process of making and drinking a cuppa can be a mindful self-care ritual.
- **Meal alone**: Solo dining can be one of midlife's pleasures and privileges.
- **Reading Snack**: Enjoy a book.
- **Shower/bath ritual**: Fill your bath with bubbles, light a candle and sit back for a self-care soak.
- **Essential oils**: Enjoy an aromatherapy snack.
- **Massage Snack**: This will relax your mind as well as your body.
- **Art Snack**: Take 5 or 10 minutes out to just doodle, draw or paint whatever you fancy.
- **Creativity Snack**: The act of being creative or artistic can leave you feeling more enthusiastic and happier that day and the next.

- **Cooking Snack**: Make your favourite meal, and cook with love.
- **Pet Snack**: Pets can reduce stress, anxiety and depression, ease loneliness, encourage exercise and playfulness, and even improve your cardiovascular health.
- **Declutter Snack**: Cleanse your environment and cleanse your mind too.
- **Gardening/Planting Snack**: This popular labour of love can provide stress relief, improve self-esteem and boost immunity, strength, heart health and brain health.
- **Sunshine Snack**: See page 305.
- **Flowers**: Buy yourself some beautiful blooms.
- **Volunteering/Giving Back Snack**: See the section on social connections starting on page 323.
- **Podcast Snack**: Tune in to your favourite podcast on your Feel Good walk, in the car or on your daily commute.
- **Smiling Snack**: See page 281.
- **Do Nothing Snack**: Yes, literally that!

Don't *find* time for the things that matter, *make* time

Mindful Minute 5.5 Breath Snack

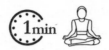

The 5.5 'coherent breathing' technique will change the way you breathe. It's the perfect breath to calm the body and mind.

This snack is perfect for those moments of overwhelm, or just to hit pause in our fast-paced lives.

Method

Breathe in for 5.5, breathe out for 5.5. As author James Nestor says, this is the most efficient breathing rhythm: 'The perfect breath is this: Breathe in for about 5.5 seconds, then exhale for 5.5 seconds. That's 5.5 breaths a minute for a total of about 5.5 litres of air.' See the section on breath, starting on page 258, for more on this.

1. Sit up straight, relax your shoulders and belly, and exhale.

2. Inhale through the nose softly for 5–6 seconds, expanding the belly as air fills the bottom of the lungs.

3. Without pausing, exhale softly through the nose for 5-6 seconds, bringing the belly in as the lungs empty.

4. Repeat 5-6 times or for one minute.

Benefits

- Calms the body and mind
- Instils a moment of peace
- Boosts mental health and mood
- Increases blood flow to the brain
- Offers the same benefits as meditation but so quickly and easily

Next steps

- I would start with a minute and build up to 5 or 10 minutes, which can give profound results.

Top tips

- Don't worry if you're a half-second off, breathing at a rate of 5 or 6 seconds – as long as the breaths are in the close range of 5.5.
- Each breath should feel like a circle. If you are having difficulty with the timing, several free apps offer timers and visual guides to breathing.
- Try to breathe through your nose, not your mouth. Nasal breathing is more efficient and has a host of benefits, so breathe through your nose whenever you can. See the Alternate Nostril Breathing Snack on page 289.

Happy
Jar Snack

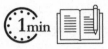

A joyful way to count your blessings, and deposit a dose of gratitude and positivity, by filling up a glass jar you can treasure and which will pick you up during any low moments.

There is no right or wrong way to fill your happy jar. The first time we tried it as a family, we started in January and aimed to do this every day in the hope that our jar would be full of 365 happy pieces to unfold at the end of the year. We didn't manage it every single day, but we still ended up with so many lovely memories to treasure.

Equipment

- A mason/glass jar (which you can decorate with stickers or photographs)
- A note pad or colourful bits of paper

Method

1. Write down one good thing that happened to you, or one thing that you are grateful for, each day of the year; fold it up and pop it in the jar.

2. At the end of the year, open the jar and reflect on all the amazing things that happened, and cherish plenty of wonderful memories.

3. Encourage your family to do the same. My boys and I have filled our happy jar with special moments, memories, accomplished goals, quotes, jokes, events, personal achievements or reminders of the simple joys in everyday life.

Benefits

- Helps you practise gratitude
- Bonds you with your loved ones
- Improves mental health
- Encourages positivity
- Shifts a negative mindset
- Improves self-esteem
- Boosts your mood

Daily Affirmation Snack

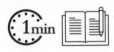

Daily affirmations are positive statements that you can recite and repeat to yourself. Sounds amazing, right?

This will help motivate you, boost your self-esteem and encourage positive changes.

Method

All you need to do is pick a phrase and repeat it to yourself.

Here are some examples to start, but you should choose ones that reflect your core personal values and really resonate with you.

- I am confident and capable at what I do.
- Today I am going to tackle everything bravely, calmly and with confidence.
- I choose to be happy.
- I believe in myself and trust my own wisdom.
- I am gifted with and surrounded by amazing friends and family.
- I accept and love myself, thoroughly and completely.
- I am resilient, strong and brave, and I can't be destroyed.

- No one but me decides how I feel.
- I choose to rise above negative feelings and ditch negative thoughts.
- When I lie down to sleep, everything is as it should be and I rest content.
- Through courage and hard work, I can achieve anything and set my mind to anything.
- I am working every day on the best me that I can be.

Benefits

- Improves mental health
- Encourages positivity
- Shifts a negative mindset
- Improves self-esteem
- Acts as a confidence booster
- Boosts your mood

―――――――

Top tips

- Try a few affirmations; make up ones for yourself and write them down as a list in your journal so you can refer to them and pick 'n' mix in future.
- If you're using a mirror or saying your affirmation to yourself, maybe place your hands on your heart as you recite it.
- Share this snack with your close family, kids or loved ones to plant the seed of gratitude. They may decide to add it to their toolkit too.

Mindful Minute Box Breath Snack

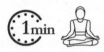

This is the best breathing technique to use in any stressful situation! It works wonders, believe me!

It's the technique I showed in my TED talk and is used by highly trained military individuals – also called 'the Navy SEAL breathing technique' – to steel their nerves and focus before entering high-pressure situations. It can also be used to return breathing to its normal rhythm after a stressful experience.

Method

Also known as the 'box breath', you can picture a box as you do this 4-4-4-4 breath, moving along its sides.

1. Sit comfortably, seated upright, with your feet on the floor.

2. Close your eyes and then breathe in through your nose while counting to four, slowly, feeling the air enter into your lungs.

3. Hold your breath while counting slowly to four.

4. Slowly exhale for 4 seconds.

5. Hold your breath while counting to four before breathing in again through your nose.

6. Repeat steps 1 to 5 at least three times.

Benefits

- Improves focus and concentration
- Relieves stress
- Reduces anxiety
- Manages pain
- Improves sleep

Next steps

- Stack on the Superbrain Snack on page 287.

_____

Top tips

- If you find the technique challenging, you can try counting to three instead of four. Once you are used to the technique, you may choose to count to five or six.
- If you're new to box breathing, it may be difficult to get the hang of it. You may also get dizzy after a few rounds, which is normal. As you practise it more often, it will improve. But if you do get dizzy, stay sitting for a minute and then resume normal breathing.

Smiling Snack

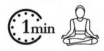 1min

Feeling down? Simply smile to release feel-good endorphins, trick your brain into happiness and boost your health. And yes, there's a science behind smiling (plus it's contagious).

Charles Darwin's facial feedback hypothesis suggested that emotions could be altered by the activity of the facial muscles. Hence why I wanted to include this free, quick trick and harness the happiness of smiling, with 'the science of smiles'. Often when I am stressed or upset, I cheer myself up by looking into the mirror and smiling. I know it sounds silly, but it works. Don't knock it until you try it!

Method

Are you smiling while you read this? Go on!

Have you ever tried to hold a pencil with your teeth? Research has shown that intentionally exercising your facial muscles (the zygomaticus major muscle and orbicularis oculi muscle) can actually make you feel better. Because this is mimicking the action of smiling.

So what is going on in our brains when we smile? Imagine you are in a pleasant situation, like bumping into an old friend on the train. When your brain feels happy, endorphins are produced and neuronal signals are transmitted to your facial muscles to trigger a smile. This is the start of the positive feedback loop of happiness. When your smiling muscles contract, they spur a powerful chemical reaction in the brain, releasing dopamine and serotonin, which can make you feel happier. Basically, when your brain feels happy, you smile; when you smile, your brain feels happier.

When you're stressed or down, go to the bathroom mirror and give yourself a smile!

Benefits

- Boosts mood
- Lowers stress
- Boosts the immune system
- Lowers blood pressure
- Lowers heart rate

Next steps

- Combine it with your morning routine, maybe a Wake-Up Stretch Snack on page 127, a breath snack or a journal snack.
- Pick a balance snack. Smile while you balance!
- Smile during any snack: the more you smile, the better!

Mindful Minute 4-6 Breath Snack

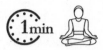

The power of a longer exhale is incredible. This trick is definitely one to put in your Feel Good toolkit before bed, or anytime you need to chill out and relax.

When we take slow, deep breaths, it elicits a state of calm and relaxation and signals our nervous system to switch from sympathetic (fight or flight) to parasympathetic mode (recover and relax).

Method

1. Simply breathe in for 4 seconds; breathe out for 6 seconds. That's it. There's no app, no special mantra or anything fancy. Just the power of your breath! Just sit down, breathe, and benefit.

2. Repeat as many times as needed. I think you will feel the benefits from just 1 minute of this intentional breathing.

Benefits

- Increases relaxation
- Instils calm

- Reduces symptoms of overwhelm, anxiety, depression, anger and confusion
- Allows you to be present
- Helps alertness
- Promotes mental fitness

Next steps

- Stack it on to the End of Day Stretch Snack on page 92, the Bed Stretch Snack on page 241, and any of the sleep tips on page 315.

Top tips

- You can do this sitting or standing; just keep your back straight, to align your diaphragm, and breathe into your belly. Perhaps place one hand on your chest and one on your stomach, to check your belly is rising.
- Count to whatever feels comfortable for you. If your exhale is longer than your inhale, it's going to help the parasympathetic nervous system to kick in, to aid rest, recovery and digestion.

Dose of Vitamin G Snack

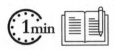

Writing down three things you're grateful for is one of the quickest ways to lift your spirits. I do this daily to get my dose of vitamin G.

Studies show that actively practising gratitude makes you happier, can help you sleep, help you de-stress, can lower your blood pressure, and has long-lasting effects on the brain – whether that's consciously thinking of what you're grateful for, or actually writing it down. Research also shows that a grateful mindset can increase the chance of you adopting healthy habits, such as exercising regularly, and result in less physical illness.

Method

Here are 3 doses/snacks for you to try out.

1. *Pen to paper*

    Write down 3 very specific things you're grateful for. Whatever you write just has to be personal and true to you. Nothing is too big or too small; it can be the simplest thing, as the act of gratitude gives everything a place. The great thing about writing it down is that this bank of gratitude is there for you to read all over again, especially when things are feeling difficult in life. Dose up on daily gratitude (vitamin G) by journaling every day – all you need is a notebook and a pen.

2. *365 days of gratitude*

    Before you go to sleep, or first thing in the morning, start the first line with a number 1 and then write something you're grateful for. Simply keep numbering and adding a daily gratitude entry, and continue for the whole year.

3. *Verbal practice*

    All you have to do is think of 3 things you're grateful for. I personally love doing this at night while I'm in bed, as I'm falling asleep. This really helps me appreciate everything I have. It helps me counteract the to-do list, alleviates any worries, and transports me away from the business of daily life, as well as putting a smile on my face before I snooze. But you could do it in the morning, and it will set you up positively for the day. Or do it at any time of the day, whenever you need a quick dose of vitamin G!

Benefits

- Helps adopt a positive outlook
- Boosts your mood
- Better mental health
- Improves sleep
- Helps reduce stress
- Boosts your brain
- Improves self-esteem and motivation

Superbrain Snack

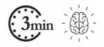

This ancient technique of squats has been found to improve mental health and alleviate brain fog – which we may battle with during menopause.

Superbrain yoga is a holistic technique used to enhance brain function, improve mood and promote health. It is particularly popular as a method of improving cognitive function and performance.

It stimulates the acupressure points in your earlobes, which sends electrical signals to the brain, thus stimulating it and boosting cognitive clarity. Plus you get all the benefits of the squat, 'king' of lower body exercises (see the Squat Snack on page 221).

Method

1. Simply cross your arms and connect your tongue to the roof of your mouth.

2. Clasp your earlobes with your opposite thumb and forefinger – right hand to the left ear and vice versa. Your left arm should be closest to your body.

3. Stand with your feet a hip width apart.

4. Inhale deeply and lower down into a squat position. Exhale as you push back up.

5. Repeat for 2–3 mins or 10–21 reps.

Refer to the Squat Snack on page 221 for squat tips.

Benefits

- Boosts brain, cognition and clarity
- Helps banish brain fog
- Improves performance
- Lowers stress
- Boosts memory and attention

Next steps

- To boost focus at work, stack this on to the Desk Reset Snack on page 76, the Desk Stretch Snack on page 160 or the Alternate Nostril Breathing Snack on page 289.

Top Tips

- Adding a rucksack as a weight is a great way to progress – but keep your hands free.

Alternate Nostril Breathing Snack

Alternate nostril breathing is a simple yet powerful technique that settles the mind, body and emotions and is perfect for the menopausal Feel Good toolkit!

In general, it's healthier to breathe through your nose instead of your mouth. That's because nose breathing is more natural and helps your body more effectively use the air you inhale. Nasal breathing could have particular benefits for people with asthma, allergies, stress, anxiety, poor exercise tolerance, poor dental health and infections, and nasal congestion, as well as snorers and those with sleep apnoea – sounds like lots of perimenopause symptoms.

Breathing through your nose may improve cognitive function, which is particularly useful for menopausal women. Breathing therapy might also be helpful to lower blood pressure and for people with cardiovascular disease (remember, it's important to reduce our risks in midlife).

Method

This method of alternate nostril breathing, Anulom Vilom, is a form of pranayama. My mum has been doing it daily for decades.

1. With your right hand, bring your index finger and middle finger to rest between your eyebrows, like an anchor.

2. Close your right nostril with your right thumb.

3. Take a deep breath through your left nostril.

4. Remove your thumb from your right nostril and close your left nostril with your ring finger.

5. Slowly exhale through your right nostril.

6. Repeat on other side. (This is one cycle.)

7. Do as many cycles of this as time allows. I recommend 5–10 cycles to hit that reset button. Build up to 5 minutes, if you have time.

Practise alternate nostril breathing regularly in order to see and maintain results.

Enjoy doing it in the morning or evening. It can also be done during the day, whenever you need to focus or relax.

Benefits

- Relaxes your body and mind
- Reduces anxiety
- Promotes overall well-being
- May help you to be more focused and aware
- Helps manage stressors in your daily life
- Makes you more mindful of the present moment

Next steps

- Follow on with your daily Dose of Vitamin G Snack on page 285 or a journal snack.
- Or add a stretch snack and/or something from the menu of self-care nibbles on page 269 for the ultimate self-care, both body and mind.

Top tips

- Ideally sit in a comfortable position, perhaps with your legs crossed.
- This is best done on an empty stomach.

3 Goals for the Day Snack

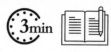

I often feel overwhelmed by my list of to-dos, so this really helps give me just 3 achievable things to tick off.

Method

Simply jot down 3 goals that you want to achieve in the day. They could be work, home or health related. You could even write one from each of these categories. There's no right or wrong.

Benefits

- Aids focus
- Reduces overwhelm
- Helps you prioritize
- Gives a sense of accomplishment when done

Next steps

- Celebrate when you've done it with a minute of star jumps or a Feel Good Hug Snack on page 80.

Write Away Your Worries Snack

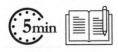

Take just 5 minutes to write away anything that's troubling or worrying you. Release and let go of it on paper to clear your mind.

Writing can be such a fabulous way to release anything that's worrying you. I know this myself! I leave a blank notebook by my bedside and often do this before bed, when my mind is congested with thoughts, actions, things I forgot to do, any troublesome moments from the day, or anything that is making me anxious (future or present). I turn to the open safe space before bedtime, in the middle of the night (if I can't sleep), or sometimes in the morning if I wake up worrying about the day ahead or have had a bad dream.

Method

This release will help you clear space for your thoughts.

1. It doesn't even have to make sense – just write it out! Get it out of your head and on to the page. Just write freely.

2. Another technique to let go is to write down literally everything that's stressing you out, and then rip it up. There, it's gone!

You may wonder why I'm recommending writing so much, rather than making notes in your phone notes app (which I often also do). There's something more effective about putting pen to paper to help alleviate stress and improve memory. See the Expressive Writing Snack on page 303.

Benefits

- Helps you clear your mind
- Encourages self-awareness
- Releases your fears, to manifest your dreams
- Declutters your mind
- Aids restful sleep
- Reduces anxiety and worry

Next steps

- If, like me, you start writing and it goes over 5 minutes, that's great. I want you to share the incredible benefits of sitting and writing for longer – often called 'expressive' writing.
- If you're struggling or not in the mood for this, gain some journaling inspiration from the quick Dose of Vitamin G Snack on page 285.

Tree Snack

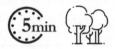

Trees are terrific. The wonder of nature and green medicine.

The benefits of forest therapy are due to airborne chemicals called phytoncides. These possess antibacterial and antifungal qualities, which plants and trees emit to protect themselves from insects and germs, but these also improve the function of our human immune system. In fact, they are so powerful that, when we breathe them in, our bodies increase the number and activity of our white blood cells – the cells we need to kill tumours, cancers and viruses in the body.

Method

Forest bathing is the therapeutic Japanese practice of *shinrin-yoku*, which is the art and science of how trees can promote health and happiness.

I love connecting with nature to boost my mood and release endorphins. I highly recommend the traditional walk in the woods. It's been my free therapy since becoming a mum and throughout perimenopause.

Benefits

- Reduces your stress levels
- Strengthens your immune and cardiovascular systems
- Boosts your energy and mood
- Can even help you lose weight
- Can help you live longer
- Reduces mental fatigue
- Boosts your natural killer white blood cells

Next steps

- If you can't get to a forest or a park, then your garden or tree-lined street will do. Studies show these produce many of the same benefits. The point is to get outside in nature and simply walk near trees. It's one of the simplest, easiest and most effective things we can do for our health. And it's free!
- Hug a tree. By simply wrapping your arms around the trunk of a tree, it releases oxytocin (to help you feel calm and emotionally bonded) as well as serotonin and dopamine (to make you happier).

Soak yourself in nature to nourish your soul

Grounding Snack

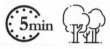

Get grounded! Simply try walking barefoot. Connect with the Earth, and boost your well-being. Such a simple, great idea.

Earthing (also known as grounding) refers to the direct skin/bodily contact with the surface of the Earth. The natural electric properties of the Earth provide many physiological benefits at the deepest level, from reducing inflammation, pain and stress to improving blood flow, energy and sleep, and generating greater well-being.

Method

Simply do your Feel Good Walk Snack on page 207 barefoot, on the grass in your garden, or play in the park without shoes, or if you're really lucky walk barefoot on a beach. I personally love walking in the sand and connecting with Mother Earth.

Or you can try swimming in natural bodies of water – oceans, lakes or rivers – as a perfect way to ground yourself. Feel the cool water, soft sand, and even slimy rocks or smooth river stones, to feel more connected to the Earth.

Benefits

- Reduces inflammation
- Shifts your nervous system into calming parasympathetic mode
- Improves wound healing
- Reduces blood pressure
- Improves muscle recovery
- Reduces pain
- Alleviates stress and depression
- Improves sleep
- Helps lower fatigue

Next steps

- Combine this with a breath snack. The Mindful Minute Box Breath Snack on page 279 is perfect for this – and maybe you can tie it into your footsteps – but feel free to pick 'n' mix.
- Add in a few moves from the Squat Snack on page 221, which you can do barefoot too.

Bird Snack

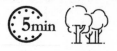

Simply listen to the birds to boost your mental health and instil positivity.

Birds appear to be a specific source of healing benefits. They are almost everywhere and provide a way to connect us to nature. Being around birds, seeing or hearing them, is associated with better mental health. (Intriguingly, birds seem to benefit healthy participants as well as people who have been diagnosed with depression.) Plus, the benefits persist well beyond your bird encounter, as the effects can last for hours after.

Method

It doesn't have to be seeing birds in real time; listening to recorded birdsong is shown to reduce feelings of anxiety and depression. So if you can't get out and about, you could even listen to a recording of birdsong through headphones to alleviate negative emotions.

Benefits

- Reduces feelings of anxiety
- Combats depression and paranoia

Train the Brain Snack

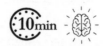

Neuroplasticity, also called brain plasticity, refers to the brain's capability to adapt and change, and is key to keeping cognitively fit.

Most of the brain's development and neuroplasticity takes place in early life, before the age of twenty-five. But, between the ages of twenty-five and sixty-five, there are still many neuroplasticity exercises you can do. This is great for us women, to keep our brains active and help banish brain fog in menopause, and reduce our risks of developing dementia and Alzheimer's.

Method

Here are some traditional ways to train your mind.

- **Learn something new**: Learn a new language or instrument, to create new neural connections. The brain loves something new and novel.
- **Play games**: Challenging your brain can improve neural pathways – try online apps, crosswords, jigsaws or sudoku puzzles, or board games with friends.
- **Change up your daily routine**: Shifting habits helps create new neural pathways. Take an alternative route

to work (preferably on foot). Stand on one foot while brushing your teeth (see the 10 Second Balance Snack on page 86).

- **Practise neurobics**: Open doors, brush your teeth, cut your veggies (carefully), carry your shopping bags or try writing – all with your non-dominant hand. Performing actions with your non-dominant hand can stimulate your brain and strengthen neural pathways, rather than allowing you to run on autopilot!
- **Use it or lose it**: Next time you go shopping, use your memory to put together your shopping list.
- **Play, sing or listen to music**: Music touches our brain, body, heart and soul. It evokes precious memories and can elicit deep emotions. Its therapeutic powers can soothe and reduce stress, or energize and invigorate. Do you remember the words to your favourite old songs?

Benefits

- Keeps your brain fit and flexible
- Ignites neuroplasticity
- Boosts your memory
- Boosts your mood with a challenge

Next steps

- Stack with other snacks, for example, a journal snack or a breath snack, or try the Social Media Snack on page 346, to give the brain some downtime to reset.

Expressive Writing Snack

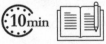

A longer invitation to write your heart out about your deepest emotions or difficult experiences. Expressive writing is healing and can help release, restore, repair and renew your mind.

As stress, anxiety and depression are so common for women in midlife, this is a great therapeutic tool to help reduce these, as well as improve our sleep, general well-being and performance, and bring us greater focus and clarity. It can help us process what we've been through, as well as assist us as we envision a path forward.

Method

1. Write about any experience that recurs in your mind – those worries that keep you up at night. The beauty of this exercise is that what may be difficult to express out loud can be given a voice through your writing.

2. Download all your thoughts and feelings, get creative, see it as me-time.

3. Sit down with your journal or a blank sheet of paper and write down your deepest emotions, in as much detail as possible. Don't hold back.

4. You don't have to be a professional writer – don't worry about grammar, spelling or sentence structure. (You can even throw it away afterwards.)

5. Simply, write your heart out!

Benefits

- Helps process experiences
- Can boost brain power
- Helps heal from trauma
- Reduces negative thoughts
- Reduces stress, anxiety and depression
- Increases resilience
- Improves sleep and performance
- Brings greater focus and clarity
- Lowers blood pressure
- Can strengthen the immune system
- Increases general well-being

Next steps

- Why not try 10 minutes? Give it a go – and if you don't like it, try something else. There are so many snacks to choose from.
- If you enjoy it, and want to write for longer, just continue.

Sunshine Snack

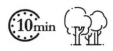

Sunlight is essential for human health and well-being, but it will also help alleviate common peri/menopausal issues like interrupted sleep, weight gain, increased stress and low mood.

Research indicates that exposure to natural light in the morning will help you sleep better. Sunshine regulates your circadian rhythm by telling your body when to increase and decrease your melatonin levels. So the more daylight exposure you can get, the better your body will become at producing melatonin when it's time to go to sleep. For more on why sleep is key to feeling good, see the section starting on page 313.

Getting outside for 30 minutes sometime between 8 a.m. and noon has also been linked to weight loss. There could be other factors to this, of course, but it seems there's a connection between sunlight in the early morning and weight loss. Studies show that morning light may also affect the hormones leptin (the satiating hormone) and ghrelin (the hunger hormone) in ways that promote a healthy bodyweight.

As the pandemic has prompted more of us to work from home, our circadian clock doesn't benefit, and we are missing out on the morning light we'd typically get from our commute into work. It's also reported that people spend about 87 per cent of their time indoors these days, so we have to make a real effort to step out into the daylight.

Method

Ideally, take a walk snack or sunshine snack outdoors in the morning (as soon as you can after waking up) and expose yourself to some rays before midday for all these incredible health benefits.

Benefits

- Improves your sleep
- Reduces stress
- Generates the production of vitamin D
- Keeps bones healthy (especially important for women in midlife and beyond)
- Reduces the risk of osteoporosis
- Helps keep the weight off
- Strengthens your immune system
- Lowers blood pressure
- Fights off depression
- Improves mental health
- Improves your alertness and energy

Next steps

- Take your journal or breath snacks outdoors. Or do your stretch and exercise snacks outdoors. Aim to spend 1 hour outside a day if you can.
- Another good time for a Feel Good walk outside is between 1 p.m. and 3 p.m. in the afternoon (when the

body produces another brief spike of melatonin). Instead of a coffee break when you start to feel sluggish in the afternoon, go outside and take a sunshine break. Leave your sunglasses off to get the full effect.

Top tips

- If you spend most of your time indoors during the day, situate yourself so you face the window and open the blinds whenever possible. If your daytime room has no window, or just a small one, add more light.
- It's worth noting that light is like a cup of coffee. It's best to minimize bright light at night, since it has the same awakening effect as in the morning – we don't want it to disrupt our sleep.

Self-care is vital to self-love

Feel Good for Life

Your fitness journey doesn't work in isolation. All three sections of this book – mind, body and life – are meant to work in harmony with each other, to support you through life's challenges and to help you thrive and be the best version of yourself. As we go through the menopause transition and think about how we can improve our long-term health, we have to adopt a 360 degree holistic, balanced approach. This book provides some tools for our physical and mental health, but these have to be supported by our lifestyle.

Sleep, food, recovery, social connections and work are also key components of the Feel Good method/toolkit. All these aspects of our life can change the way we feel, and can play a big part in our menopause journey and longer-term health. It's like a cycle; all of them are components that complement each other and work best together.

I know how I feel if I haven't had a good night's sleep, for example, and it affects my work, my relationships and social skills, the food I eat and my motivation to move. Similarly, I recall multiple scenarios at work that used to affect my self-esteem, trigger anxiety or disrupt my sleep and diminish my overall zest for life. This book provides flavoursome snacks to give you tools to help with these core aspects of your life.

Let's discuss some of the main areas of our lives and see how we can invest in them to feel good in midlife, menopause and beyond. Share these ideas with your colleagues, friends, online communities or social communities (you can tag me) and also with your daughters (so they are prepared and fully equipped too).

I truly want you to Feel Good for life!

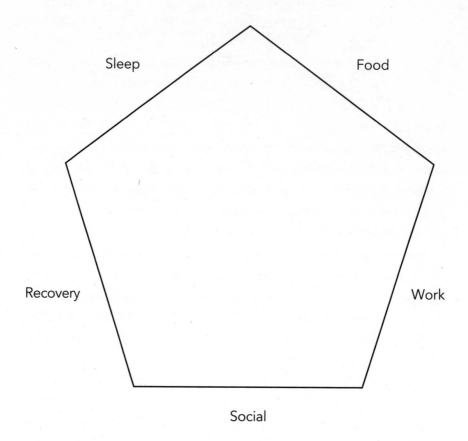

Sleep

Food

Recovery

Work

Social

Sleep

So many women I know struggle with their sleep, especially in midlife. It's a fact that insomnia is almost twice as common in women as in men. Much of this has to do with hormones, from puberty and menstruation to pregnancy, post-partum and menopause. But some of it has to do with the ebbs and flows of a woman's life.

Women are also at increased risk of experiencing certain mental health conditions, such as anxiety and depression, which can exacerbate sleep issues. According to the National Sleep Foundation around 61 per cent of menopausal women have sleep problems. This is because the fall in oestrogen and progesterone can affect the body's temperature control, leading to symptoms like hot flushes and night sweats.

Insomnia and broken sleep can make daily life difficult – impacting both your physical and mental well-being. The hormonal roller coaster can leave you feeling fatigued and deflated, which is not conducive to exercising or eating well.

We cannot ignore the importance of getting enough sleep, as exercise and sleep have a bidirectional relationship. The more regularly you exercise, the better your sleep, and vice versa. There is solid evidence that exercise does, in fact, help you fall asleep more quickly and improves sleep quality.

Exercise helps sleep by boosting our metabolism, increasing the by-product called adenosine and the drive to sleep. It increases the speed at which we fall asleep and the depth of sleep. It's also fantastic at mopping up the stress hormones running around our system, to promote better sleep as well.

Why is sleep so important?

Sleep is such an important building block for our health and well-being and is central for our fitness too. When we exercise, we are applying physical stress to the body, and muscles get stronger in the period after the workout when the body is repairing the 'damage'. Sleep is a vital function of the body that helps the mind and body to rejuvenate and recover. It is even more important for more active people, as it helps heal and repair muscles, blood vessels and the heart (reducing the risk of kidney and cardiovascular disease, obesity, diabetes, high blood pressure and strokes). Importantly, allowing your body to recover properly makes it easier to be more active the next day.

The sweet spot for adults is to get 7–8 hours of sleep per night. Here are some compelling reasons why hitting the sack is just as important as hitting that workout!

- Sleeping less than 8 hours increases the stress hormone cortisol, which causes you to store more fat in your stomach.
- Inadequate sleep (i.e. less than 6 hours) can increase your calorie intake by 30 per cent, which leads to weight gain.
- Anabolic growth hormone is released when you sleep, contributing to muscle growth and recovery.

Top tips to help you feel good with sleep

1. **Exercise regularly**: Keep snacking on exercise throughout the day (just not within 2 hours of bedtime).
2. **Follow a consistent routine**: Keep regular sleep hours.
3. **Manage the light you see**: Avoid screens or use amber glasses; employ night-time mode on your devices to minimize blue light exposure in the evenings. Ideally, keep the hour before bed screen-free.
4. **Create a restful environment**: Dim the lights and make your bed a comfy sanctuary. Keep your room temperature cool and wear suitable breathable fabrics, especially if you get hot flushes or night sweats (natural fibres like cotton, silk, bamboo, merino wool are best, and layering could be the way forward).
5. **Cut down on caffeine**: And no coffee after 2 p.m. as it stays in your system longer than you think.
6. **Write away your worries**: Check out the snacks with the journal icon.
7. **Don't eat a heavy meal too late in the day**: Perhaps try time-restricted eating (see the section 'Top tips to help you feel good with food' on page 354).
8. **Expose yourself to daylight when you wake up**: Ideally, go for a Feel Good Walk Snack on page 207, outdoors in the morning, to help produce melatonin and reset your circadian rhythm (your body's inbuilt clock). Or enjoy a Sunshine Snack on page 305.

9. **Relax**: Have a hot shower or bath or take time to relax/read/treat yourself to some self-care before bed. See the menu of self-care nibbles on page 269.

10. **Unwind with a gentle stretch and breath flow**: I keep a yoga mat at the end of my bed for a sleep stretch snack every night (try the End of Day Stretch Snack on page 92). Tie it in with a breath snack (look out for the breath icon) like the Mindful Minute 4-6 Breath Snack on page 283.

Recovery

Life isn't always perfect, and on the days when I haven't managed to get a good night's sleep or I've not been able to follow a consistent routine, I highly recommend taking a Nap Snack (see page 344). In fact, it's said to be more beneficial than trying to get an extra 30 minutes of sleep during the night and may produce the same benefits as a full night of sleep. So instead of being anxious – stressing, tossing and turning and worrying in the middle of the night – just try this hack.

Just like sleep, it's important to build in recovery time. When it comes to improving your fitness and building muscle, it's the time you spend outside of exercising when the magic really happens. When you work out, you create micro-tears in your muscle fibres. After each session, your body rebuilds those damaged muscle fibres so they are stronger than before. Your body needs days off to repair, recover and rest – without them, you miss out on the muscle-making magic. Taking rest days is a way to allow us to ensure that we can continuously do the activity we love.

Regardless of one's fitness level, exercise for women in their forties and beyond is somewhat different than for those in their twenties and thirties. Physical changes, such as slower metabolism, hormonal changes during perimenopause and menopause, and the higher risk of developing cardiac and bone issues in midlife, all make it important to take a closer look at best practices for fitness. Midlife is the time to move, strengthen muscles and stretch more. This is a time to be kind to our bodies too and give ourselves ample time and tools to aid with recovery. As we age, we need to ensure we rest and recover alongside physical activity.

The exact amount of rest and recovery time required depends on your individual fitness levels and the type of exercise you're doing. After the age of fifty, you may need more recovery time because your muscle tissues take longer to heal. I advise you to listen to your body, and if you need an extra day off between strength snacks, take it.

Of course, rest days don't have to mean sitting on the couch all day. An active recovery day could include a leisurely Feel Good walk, a stretch or a restorative mobility snack. Or you can pick something you enjoy doing that feels restful from the menu of recovery nibbles below.

Recovery nibbles

- **Magnesium**: This is a powerful relaxation mineral for muscles and the nervous system, and it can also aid sleep – all of which are great for recovery. I know many women in midlife who benefit from taking a supplement regularly.
- **Stretching**: This will reduce the muscle soreness you sometimes experience. It will lengthen the muscles and aid recovery (look for the stretch icon).
- **Breath work**: Working out elevates your heart rate and activates your fight-or-flight response. Calm your body and give it time to get back to that 'rest and digest' state by doing some mindful breath snacks (look for the breath icon).
- **Stay hydrated**: Water supports the delivery of nutrients throughout your body and literally every metabolic process. Aim for 1.5 to 2.5 litres per day. I suggest drinking a glass on waking, and then 1–2 glasses before each meal, or sip a bottle throughout the day, so you aim

for 7–8 glasses. (This will keep you active too, as you'll need to keep getting up to go to the bathroom!)

- **Massage**: Traditional hands-on massage is proven to speed up recovery and can help prevent delayed onset muscle soreness (DOMS). But not everyone can do this, due to time or financial constraints, so there are self-massage tools and techniques you can use to do a pretty good job yourself. For example, foam rolling is an effective tool to add to your warm-up or cool-down. It can help relieve inflammation, muscle tightness and soreness, and increase the range of motion in your joints. It can also help break down scar tissue that may have developed in the muscles and stretch connective tissues to help circulation.
- **Sleep**: Sleep is an under-appreciated part of muscle recovery. Deep sleep triggers the release of a hormone that boosts muscle mass and helps repair cells and tissues. Check out my sleep tips on page 315 and remember, if you are struggling, treat yourself to a Nap Snack on page 344.
- **Protein**: Keep up a well-balanced diet – fuelling up on protein, which helps you rebuild muscles, and carbohydrates, which you need in order to replenish your glycogen stores and aid recovery. I recommend having protein regularly throughout the day with each meal (see more in the section on food, starting on page 352).
- **Keep moving**: An active recovery will keep the blood flowing and circulating, make sure nutrients are delivered to your muscles, and help your muscles get rid of waste. Continued movement also helps your body process lactic acid. Try a short Feel Good Walk Snack on page 207 or the Yoga Balance Snack on page 140. Or try the Seated Circulation Snack on page 183 for some easy,

gentle movements. Remember, motion is lotion for your muscles and joints.

- **Listen to your body:** If your muscles are really sore and tired, it's not worth pushing through. Don't get discouraged if you need an extra day or two to recover and have to cut one of your planned workouts. A little soreness is okay, but if you're so sore that you hurt during everyday activities, that's a sign you need to scale back, either in intensity or in the number of days. Rest and recovery are essential for getting stronger and maintaining physical health as you age, so don't be afraid to do more of it, if that's what your body is asking for.

Hot and cold exposure

The health benefits of cold and heat are huge for us women, especially when experiencing menopausal symptoms, as they include increased metabolism, improved immunity, lowered insulin resistance, as well as the potential to reduce excess weight and ease muscle pain.

There is a growing body of research and increased interest in the latest popular trends in cold and heat therapies, but many cultures have been doing it for thousands of years, knowing that exposure to different temperatures is good for us. A study in 2021 has discovered the minimum threshold – or the sweet spot – for cold and heat exposure in order to obtain health benefits. It says you only need 11 minutes cold and 57 minutes heat exposure per week.

Brown fat activation is a key factor in the health benefits of cold water immersion and heat exposure. Brown fat is a magical type of healthy fat stored around the spine that acts as our body's temperature regulator. It boosts metabolism and can even aid the regulation of blood sugar and help weight control.

The study also supports the science of micro-stressing the body – meaning that health benefits are obtained by small doses of healthy stress, i.e. cold and heat. Healthy stress strengthens the cells and the mind. Overdoing stressors – or being chronically stressed – ages the cells, causes inflammation and an overwhelmed nervous system. This fits so well with my snacking concept – and with everything in life. See the Cold Water Snack on page 338 and the Heat Snack on page 341. Start off small, and aim to build up to the recommended times.

The scientific research concludes that it's optimal to end sauna routines in the cold (to force the body to activate more brown fat). I know that may not be what you want to hear!

Social

Social media and social connections

Human beings are social creatures, and we need the companionship of others to thrive in life. The strength of our connections has a huge impact on our mental health and happiness. Being socially connected to others can ease stress, anxiety and depression, boost self-worth, provide comfort and joy, prevent loneliness, and even add years to your life. On the flip side, lacking strong social connections can pose a serious risk to your mental and emotional health.

In today's world, many of us rely on social media platforms to find and connect with each other. While each has its benefits, it's important to remember that social media can never be a replacement for real-world human connection. It requires in-person contact with others to trigger the hormones that alleviate stress and make you feel happier, healthier and more positive.

On average we spend two and a half hours on social media each day. That's the same amount of time as the government guidelines ask us to spend on doing exercise in a week. That's also 15 per cent of your waking life! Two in five adults grab their phone within 5 minutes of waking up, rising to 65 per cent for the under thirty-fives. I'm a culprit of this myself.

I never planned on being on social media. Before my account became public, in September 2019, I had 600 followers (all friends and family, in typical South Asian large community style). Like most of us, social media, at its inception, was harmless fun. I never imagined my exercise snacks and workouts would be viewed by more than the people who knew me, let alone saw myself becoming a content creator (I still don't feel comfortable calling myself this, or an 'influencer'), and especially not in my forties! Social media has been very positive for me and allows me to share my message, to reach people globally and help as many as I can.

However, social media can impact our sleep, worsen anxiety and depression, instil worries about body image, and heighten our fear of missing out. Ironically, for a technology that's designed to bring people closer together, for many of us, spending too much time engaging with social media can actually make us feel more lonely and isolated – and exacerbate mental health problems such as anxiety and depression.

We also know that much of social media is not real life, it's a curated and selective sample of what's actually going on in the world. No one's life is ever as perfect as it seems on social media. Everyone has challenges and issues behind closed doors. I try to keep my feed as real as possible when it comes to my journey – I've cried, been open about my struggles, and I don't use filters. I am protective of my family, as most mothers are. We all deal with heartache, self-doubt, private issues and disappointment, even if we choose not to share it online. My advice is to curate your feed and follow positive pages on your favourite social media platforms, to reshape your personal algorithm. It's the same with all screens, even TV or Netflix, so carve out time for shows that make you feel good.

Social media platforms are designed to share your attention, keep you online, and have you repeatedly checking your screen for updates. It's addictive, and that's how the companies make money. When you receive a like, a share, or a favourable reaction to a post, it can trigger the release of a dopamine hit in the brain – the feel-good 'reward' chemical.

It's safe to say screens are here to stay, they are an integral part of our daily lives, and it's how we consume most of our information. For all the downsides, there are so many positives with social media. Like being able to communicate and stay up to date with family and friends around the world; in terms of combating loneliness; networking and finding new friends and being part of a community with similar interests; promoting worthwhile causes; support during tough times; a great outlet for your creativity and expression; sources of information and learning. I can definitely relate and say that my platforms have enabled me to help and reach out to people I never imagined connecting with. And the benefits have always outweighed the times I may have experienced digital overwhelm or overload.

Social snacking

Social media is a great tool for facilitating connections but we all need the real, face-to-face company of others in order to be happy and healthy. It's dangerous when we start prioritizing online friendships over in-real-life or face-to-face connections. When it comes to staying in touch with people, we could all put a little more effort into it these days. Me included! The amount of mental energy we give our phones, specifically social media, could be put to much better use.

During my social media snacks (see page 346) and Feel Good walks, I tend to call my family and friends, just to see how they are doing for 10 minutes. You could even pick up the old tradition of pen-palling, but do it over email with long-distance friends.

During menopause, loss of confidence, anxiety and fatigue can stop you from wanting to socialize or see friends. I know many women feel more isolated and withdraw from life. I do try to spend more time in person connecting with people. Everyone is so busy nowadays, but it's important to still make an effort. If you see exercise as a way to connect with other women who can relate, support and understand, you'll find that movement will have a positive effect on how you're feeling. Go for a walk rather than a drink! Walking and talking is a great way to socialize – it's great for your physical health but it also deepens your connections with people. (And it usually means you're taking a social media snack break too – so it's a win-win!) I often walk to dinner with a friend – and back if we can too.

Group exercise classes, or doing exercise with a friend, is a great way to build connection, friendships, motivation and share a common goal.

Researchers have found that social laughter releases endorphins (feel-good hormones) in our brains. Laugh with your friends, and not only will you benefit from the giggles, but laughing can strengthen your relationships! Laughter is truly the best medicine.

On the flip side it's also important to learn to say no and to prioritize where you spend your precious time and energy – and who with! Rather than the usual FOMO (fear of missing out), exacerbated by social media, let's flip it to JOMO (the joy of missing out). Don't stress when friends hang out without you, there will be other chances. Really enjoy the special moments with your closest loved ones, and value them fully, with gratitude. We can't say yes to everything. Some boundaries are good and healthy.

Friendship in midlife and beyond

This leads me to touch on an important topic I've discussed with friends and observed with many women in midlife. Who are your true friends? Who is your tribe? What is real friendship these days?

According to Harvard Health Publishing, people who have successful and fulfilling relationships are happier, have fewer health problems and increased longevity.

Do you believe in the saying, 'You are the sum of who you surround yourself with'?

I remember my mum telling me in my twenties, when I had hundreds of friends, from university, work and socially, 'Lavina, one day you'll be able to count your true friends on your two hands.' I didn't believe her at the time, but she's so right!

How many of us have experienced toxic friendships? I think it's important to acknowledge that this happens and that you can let go when you need to. I bet we all have people in our lives who leave us feeling miserable and drained of energy – especially through challenging phases of our lives, like perimenopause and menopause, which are hard enough already. It's important to avoid having toxic energy in your life, especially if you want to maintain good health.

One study by researchers at the University of Arizona believes stress causes fluctuations of hormones, which can result in loss of bone density – leaving women vulnerable to breaks from even minor falls. They found that bone loss is among the physiological stress responses more strongly related to the *quality* of social relationships than the *quantity*. This was because stress can cause fluctuating levels of hormones including cortisol, thyroid hormones, growth hormones and glucocorticoids, which have an impact on bones. Some 60 per cent of elderly people who suffer a fracture never regain their independence.

I think it's important to recognize that the so-called 'midlife crisis' for many women is not a crisis at all. Rather, it is a point in their lives, a period of self-discovery and growth, when they finally figure out who they are, identify what they have been putting up with for years, resulting in a newfound sense of clarity and happiness. They may leave unfulfilling careers, end toxic relationships, or pursue passions they have long ignored. As women reach midlife, they begin to see through these societal expectations and start to prioritize their own needs and desires. I think we start to care less about what others think and focus more on what brings us joy and fulfilment. We can shed things that have held us back for years, and embrace midlife as a time of liberation and empowerment.

It's important to make ourselves happy by surrounding ourselves with positive people. When we choose to associate with positive people, we tend to become happier and brighter and enjoy better lives. In fact, one study urges us to prioritize our midlife mates for our health. University of Queensland research has found that women who have quality relationships in their forties and fifties are less likely to develop multiple chronic conditions in older age. Between simultaneously caring for your elders and the younger generations, and managing your peri/menopause, catching up with pals can feel like something you don't have time for. The study showed that those women who were 'dissatisfied' with their relationships were more than twice as likely to develop conditions like type 2 diabetes, arthritis, heart disease or asthma.

Research shows that having a strong social life seems to be protective against cognitive decline. In fact, studies have found that people with more positive social relationships than their peers have better brainpower as they age.

Find and surround yourself with friends who make you feel good. It's hard to find, I know! Ones who are there to support you through the good and the bad times, without jealousy. My inner circle of friends are genuinely happy to see me happy. They don't get jealous if I'm successful; they encourage me. They don't say horrible things about me behind my back; they say kind, loving things. They understand I'm not perfect and forgive me for my flaws. They make me laugh, and they enjoy seeing me happy. It doesn't matter if we haven't met or spoken every week, we pick up where we left off. There are no grudges. This is what true friendship should be about. That's why it's so important to forgive, love, and move on from friendships if and when you have to. We all deserve to be happy, and we have the power to make it happen.

Strong social connections help us live longer and lead healthier lives

Numerous studies provide evidence that an active social life can help you live longer. For example, research about an unusually long-living population on the island of Sardinia, in Italy, has shown that strong ties to family and friends, along with frequent physical activity, may contribute to their longevity.

Just as we plan our exercise snacks it's equally important to do social snacking and spend quality time with friends and family. In addition, think about how to incorporate kindness into your routine, whether that's through formal volunteering or more informal random acts of kindness, as these are powerful ways to boost social connections. In one study, elderly people who volunteered were 44 per cent less likely to die over the course of a 5 year study. So prioritize social engagements in your own life, and make it a healthy habit, just as important as physical exercise.

Social nibbles

Here are some ideas to get you socializing. It's a great page to screenshot and share with your friends, loved ones and parents.

- Join a group exercise class.
- Walk and talk with a friend.
- Call a friend (rather than messaging them).
- Do an exercise snack with a friend and set up a weekly challenge so you stay in touch.

- Volunteer with an organization.
- Join a fitness community online.
- Join a local activity like Parkrun.
- Do some community work.
- Join a charity fitness fundraiser.
- Join my Feel Good community – online workouts.
- Spend more time with family and friends.
- Turn a virtual/phone meeting into a face-to-face meet-up.
- Join a new class or start a new hobby.
- Start up a monthly menopause coffee morning.
- Set up a recurring diary invite with your best friends.
- Have 'bring a dish' get-togethers at different friends' houses.

Work

There are so many benefits of workplace wellness – building in exercise snacks and frequently doing workday exercise – and they have a ripple effect on other areas of life, including:

- mental health benefits
- reducing stress levels and anxiety
- increasing productivity and creativity
- fewer sick days due to stress, illness or pain
- improved energy, sleep, creativity, mood
- stronger immune system and a reduced risk of chronic illness.

Employers should adapt working policies to target physical activity, stress and diet. We should make exercise compulsory and a normal part of the day at work. The benefits have long been known: exercise during the day and you'll look better, feel better and even work better. Physical activity boosts workplace morale and helps keep you mentally healthier. The cognitive outcomes at work of increased productivity, better focus and a clearer mind should not be underestimated as quick wins and benefits to employers. It's hard to maintain a robust team if people are leaving, or dying of preventable diseases.

People who exercise during the day find they get more work done and take fewer sick days. Plus, it's good for mental health, providing a stress-free getaway from the daily typhoon of meetings and emails. In essence, happier employees equal a happier company!

Why this subject matters to me

I worked in the corporate world in my twenties, in a role with a lot of responsibility, managing teams onshore and offshore, as a female in an environment dominated by men, most of whom were older than me. So I love going into workplaces today with my corporate hat on!

I always put myself in women's shoes when I consult for workplaces and deliver keynote speeches or my Feel Good interactive workshops. I try to imagine what Lavina in her forties would feel like in a high-powered role, combined with juggling the demands of a busy family, with home responsibilities, family obligations, caring for my parents and children . . . let alone dealing with sleep disruptions, anxiety, brain fog, heavy and irregular periods, or any of the typical peri/menopausal symptoms. Imagine if I forgot my words or lost my train of thought when delivering speeches to my teams and presentations to clients, or even negotiating contracts. Imagine if I had a male boss and had to tell him my periods were so heavy that I couldn't get to work, or that I felt like I was losing my mind but didn't want my upcoming promotion or performance review to be affected, let alone my colleagues finding out how I really felt.

Women's health in the workplace

A Menopause and the Workplace report by the Fawcett Society shows that 1 in 10 women who worked during the menopause have left a job as a result of their symptoms, and 1 in 4 are contemplating leaving. Women leaders are leaving at the fastest rate for 10 years. Women, and particularly women of colour, are leaving the workforce at a record rate, and yet all the evidence is that a diverse workforce functions better.

The workplace and the economy cannot afford to lose these highly talented women who are at the peak of their game. Retaining this high-performing talent is now a business imperative and offers a competitive advantage. Corporates with women forming more than 25 per cent of their executive committee saw a profit margin of 16 per cent – more than 10 times higher than those with no female board members.

Women's health needs to be prioritized, and women need to be supported by their workplace through every stage of their careers – from menstruation, to motherhood, to menopause. That's why it's so important that we ensure workplaces have women's health high on their agenda.

Alongside the challenges of midlife and how companies can better support their staff, the other area which really concerns me in terms of workplace wellness is the lack of physical movement.

The problem with modern life and work

The big issue, as I see it, is how much time we spend sitting. Research into current levels of sedentary behaviour is limited, but we know that adults of working age in England average about 9.5 hours per day of sedentary time. Between the ages of sixty-five and seventy-four, sedentary time in both men and women increases to 10 hours per day or more. By the age of seventy-five plus, people are sedentary for 11 hours per day.

Sedentary behaviour is increasingly common in a society where many of us do desk jobs, travel in motor vehicles and spend leisure time in front of technology, computers and televisions. It also increases with age, particularly when ill health is a factor.

People who spend long periods of time sitting have been found to have higher rates of diabetes, cardiovascular disease and death from all causes (even if you're not overweight). Sitting for long periods is also associated with poor mental health, such as depression. Although it can be difficult to separate cause and effect, on the whole, people feel their minds work better when they sit less.

I see two issues when it comes to sitting.

- Firstly, how long do you sit for throughout the day? We want to reduce that time.
- The second, just as important, question is how often do you break up that sitting? We need to get up frequently and break up those long periods of sitting.

A key takeaway I want you to remember from this book is that most of us could benefit from spending less time sitting – and that applies even if you're keeping active! In fact, more and more evidence is emerging that even if you exercise regularly, spending a lot of time sitting down can be bad for you (see 'Sit less, move more' on page 35). There's no point doing your exercise for an hour in the morning, if you're going to sit for the rest of the day. You may feel good that you've worked out, but then you simply sit: on your commute straight to your desk at work, in meetings with minimal breaks, then eat your meals and sit again, have dinner and just sit on the sofa until bedtime.

This is a very common pattern and, unfortunately, hybrid working post-pandemic has exacerbated this for typical office workers. Have you counted how many hours a day you are sitting on back-to-back Zoom or virtual meetings? Don't get me wrong, there are so many benefits to hybrid working, but I guarantee you're sitting for longer periods when you're working from home. Apart from going to the fridge for food snacks, or taking bathroom breaks, you probably don't tend to move that much.

Take a break

Research has found that taking a break can be very beneficial for you and your work. Taking breaks has been shown to
be important in recovering from stress, which can, in turn,
improve your performance. Recovering from work stress can
restore energy and mental resources, and decrease the development of fatigue, sleep disorders and cardiovascular disease.

Taking a break from making decisions within work allows
employees to refuel, so they make better decisions than they
would without a break. Breaks improve employees' quality
of work, thus benefiting the organization, supervisors and
employees alike.

Research has also found it is important to take mini-breaks
throughout the working day, as they help to support your
well-being and increase productivity. Employees who step
away from work for a few minutes increase their productivity
and creativity, their job satisfaction, their mental health and
well-being, and they feel more valued by their supervisor and
organization. Overall, they feel more engaged in their work.

Exercise snacking is the perfect solution

This has been confirmed by the numerous companies I've held 'snacking workshops' for, and in the messages I've received from employees and managers who have started using my tips in their teams.

Doing some movement in short breaks from work is so beneficial. And the beauty of exercise snacking is that you don't need to have a fancy gym in your office. These are small ways of weaving exercise into your work day, and there are movement opportunities everywhere.

Work nibbles

Here are some of my top tips to get you thinking about how you can stay active and move more at work. Pick a few and write them out as your snack-size work goals.

- Diarize your workouts/snacks like you would a meeting, so you're more likely to commit to them.
- 'Snack' on exercise and treat your body and mind to bite-size amounts throughout the day.
- Set an alarm every hour (ideally every half-hour) to get up and move for 3 minutes.
- If you're working from home, fake your commute and use the time you would have walked to the station, or from the carpark to the office, as a Feel Good Walk Snack (see page 207).
    - If you're going by train/bus, get off a stop earlier on your commute and walk, cycle or run one stop (or stand if stuck on public transport).

- ○ If you're driving your car, park as far away as possible and walk that extra distance.
- ○ Turn a phone meeting into a walking meeting, or go across to talk to a colleague rather than send an email.
- ○ If you're going out to get your lunch, try a new shop further away. Get those extra little steps in without even thinking about it.
- Go for a 10 minute Feel Good Walk Snack after each meal, especially breakfast and lunchtime, so you get in some early daylight.
- If you're stuck in virtual meetings, turn your camera off and do some chair-based stretches or mobility drills, like the 1 minute Tech Neck Stretch on page 78, the 5 minute Desk Stretch Snack on page 160 or the 5 minute Seated Circulation Snack on page 183.

Cold Water Snack

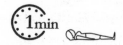

The goal is to immerse yourself in cold water for a duration of 1–2 minutes per session, with a recommended maximum of 11 minutes per week.

Cold water provides incredible benefits for your health and well-being. It can help you reduce muscle soreness (great for menopausal aches and pains), cool you down after exercise (and hot flushes), boost your immune system and metabolism, and even improve your mood (perfect for those times when you are battling with hormones and life). Just a brief immersion in cold water – for example, a blast at the end of your shower – is ideal to reap these benefits.

Method

There are several ways to try cold water exposure.

- **Cold shower**: Even just a cooler blast at the end of your normal shower is a very effective place to start. Start with 5 seconds and build up to the goal of 60–90 seconds.

You'll get a big burst of energy as your body tries to conserve heat and kicks your circulation into gear. One study found that cold showers help release endorphins, which could have an antidepressant effect.

- **Plunge pool or ice bath**: If you're a little more daring, fill your bath with cold water and add some ice. Immerse yourself for up to 5 minutes. Build up to this gradually, and use deep breathing techniques.
- **Cold water swimming**: In lakes, outdoor pools or the sea.

Benefits

- Increases metabolism
- Boosts immunity and the longevity of your cells
- Lowers insulin resistance
- Eases muscle and joint pain
- Quickens recovery after exercise
- Boosts circulation
- Protects against obesity and cardiovascular disease
- Reduces stress and anxiety
- Improves mood and happiness

Top tips

- Take time to acclimatize yourself before you take the cold plunge.
- Once you're ready for a dip, step carefully into the tub, barrel or natural body of water, and slowly lower yourself until you're submerged from the neck down. You can also target a specific region of the body. For example,

only sit in water high enough to cover the legs, to boost recovery following an intense lower-body strength snack or walking session.

- Get out if you start to shake or shiver. That's your body telling you that you've reached your maximum time for the day.

Heat Snack

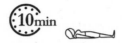

Health-giving brown fat is activated by heat as well as cold. So treat yourself to some post-workout heat, perhaps from a hot tub or sauna.

A study by Dr Susanna Søberg recommends 57 minutes per week. The ideal length of each sauna is 10–15 minutes to get profound health benefits.

Research finds that 2–3 sauna days per week reduces your risk of dying by 24 per cent. A study of more than 2,000 people over a period of 20 years found that using the sauna 4–7 times a week was associated with a 40 per cent decrease in death from all causes (compared to only one sauna session per week).

Not only does the sauna support your mental well-being but it can also help you achieve your physical fitness goals. Increased blood flow helps remove the waste products and lactic acid that accumulate during exercise, and transports nutrients and healing cells to the damaged muscles to help them recover. It may boost the release of growth hormone, which plays a key role in stimulating muscle growth, strengthening bones, repairing tissue and increasing metabolism.

Method

If you have access to a sauna, aim for 10 minutes each time.

The goal is a total of 57 minutes split up over 2-4 days, which would correspond to short bursts of 10 to 15 minutes per session.

Here are some alternatives, if you don't have access to a sauna or hot tub.

- Try some hot water therapy with a relaxing soak in your bath tub. Add some magnesium or Epsom salts to soothe aches and pains, ease muscles and draw out impurities.
- If you are on holiday or by the sea in summer, a swim in warm seawater is also fabulous. It increases circulation, eases pain or stiffness, and restores natural minerals in the body.
- Swimming in a warm indoor pool is also gentle on the joints, and the weightlessness of water has a calming effect on the mind and body.
- A hot shower will also do, and is a way to access controlled deliberate exposure to heat.

Benefits

- Improves heart rate
- Increases blood flow
- Can improve cardiovascular health
- Reduces the likelihood of developing dementia or Alzheimer's

- Improves stress response and overall health
- Reduces muscle soreness (great for menopause)
- Reduces chronic pain
- Improves heart health
- Increases metabolism
- Alleviates stress and decreases cortisol levels
- Provides me-time – relaxing, calming and a form of self-care
- Boosts mood

Next steps

- Start snacking on the sauna!
- Start slow, using cooler temperatures that don't significantly increase the heart rate.
- Hyperthermia (abnormally high body temperature) and dehydration are always possible, so proceed with caution.
- If you have any doubts, don't forget to check with a medical professional before going into the sauna for the first time.

Top tips

- As with all the snacks, listen to your body and build up gradually.
- Stay hydrated before and after.
- Using the sauna during the afternoon/evening will help match your body's natural cooling with the 'post-cooling sauna effect', in order to aid falling asleep at night.

Nap Snack

Midlife worries, tasks, hot flushes and night sweats can affect our sleep, but a nap can really work wonders.

I know many of us women struggle with sleep. It's stressful and lonely lying awake at night, desperately wishing for elusive sleep, and dealing with exhaustion the next day. In the ideal world we'd get a good night's sleep. But even if we do, many of us feel the afternoon slump after about 8 hours of our normal daytime activities.

Research shows that a nap can make you more energized, alert, reduce stress, improve cognitive function, strengthen your memory, boost your mood and even improve your health. In fact, a study shows that people who napped 1–2 times a week were 48 per cent less likely to have cardiovascular problems such as heart attack, stroke or heart failure, after an average 5 years of follow-up, compared to those who did not nap at all.

Method

Many say the ideal time to have a nap snack is after lunch and before 3 p.m. – not too late or long, so that your night-time sleep doesn't suffer.

Experts advise to keep the nap between 15 and 30 minutes. Longer naps get you into deeper phases of sleep, which are harder to awaken from and make you feel groggy.

Even closing your eyes for 5 minutes has benefits in reducing stress and helping you relax, as well as giving you more energy to complete the tasks of your day. However, a nap of 10 minutes produces immediate benefits and is the most recuperative duration, though many experts recommend 10–20 minutes to provide the best results. Test them out, by all means, and find that sweet spot. Just remember to set an alarm – or two!

Benefits

- Improves mental clarity and focus
- Boosts memory and cognitive function
- Increases energy and alertness
- Reduce levels of stress and anxiety
- Boosts your mood
- Resets your nervous system
- Reduces the risks of cardiovascular health issues, which is important for women in midlife and beyond

Top tips

- The Wake-Up Stretch Snack on page 127 is perfect after your Nap Snack.
- A HIIT Snack on page 97, even just 1 minute, or a cold shower on page 338, is also great to wake you up.

Social Media Snack

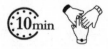

It's really important to constantly examine and re-evaluate your online habits and find a healthy balance that works for you. I have been trying to do the same, especially when writing this book.

How often do you reach for the phone first thing in the morning and check your messages, apps and notifications? How often when you're on holiday or at a family occasion are you more concerned about taking the perfect picture than enjoying yourself? How often are you locked in an internet argument or viral trend? Try the Bergen Social Media Addiction scale; simply google it and see where you stand in minutes!

Studies show that just being more mindful of your social media use can have beneficial effects on your mood and focus. There has been a recent trend of people consciously reducing their social media use to protect their mental well-being.

I'm not suggesting going cold turkey, doing a full detox and deleting all your social media accounts to experience the benefits of avoiding social media. A social media snacking approach may just be enough for you if you're experiencing the anxiety and stress that often comes with too much social media use.

Method

Here are a few ways/tips to do a social media snack.

- Resist the urge to check your social media first thing in the morning or last thing before bed.
- Turn your phone off one hour earlier. Don't bring your phone or tablet to bed. Turn devices off and leave them in another room overnight to charge.
- Spend at least one hour a day without your phone. Switch it to airplane mode, or put it in a different room. Lock it in a drawer, then try not to use it during that time.
- Turn off your notifications (as many as possible) to help you regain control of your time and focus.
- Move apps you struggle to resist away from your main screen. If you compulsively check your phone every few minutes, wean yourself off by limiting your checks to once every 15 minutes. Then once every 30 minutes, then once an hour.
- Set time slots/blocks in the diary when you are allowed to scroll. Diarize social media check windows. (Use the pomodoro working technique of 25 minutes focused work and then 5 minutes to snack on socials.)
- Turn off your phone (or do not disturb) at certain times of the day, such as when you're driving, in a meeting, doing an exercise snack, having dinner, spending time with offline friends, or playing with your kids or grandkids. Try not taking your phone with you to the bathroom.
- If you're struggling still, try an app blocker, or block off part of your screen, to curb those impulses.
- If you need to, then go off the grid for a day or a few. I did this when writing the book so I had the headspace and focus. It's amazing how much time it gave me. It

wasn't easy, and I really had to resist the urge to open my social media apps! After a day I felt really cleansed and rather than having FOMO, I felt quite refreshingly free and enjoyed some JOMO (see page 326).

- A tougher measure is to remove social media apps from your phone entirely, so you can only check them from your tablet or computer. If this sounds like too drastic a step, try removing one social media app at a time to see how much you really miss it.

Benefits

- More in the present
- Fewer distractions
- Downtime for the brain and mind
- Helps foster healthy relationships with technology
- Reduces stress and anxiety levels
- Boosts concentration and focus
- Boosts mood
- Less comparison, less FOMO
- Gives the eyes a rest

Next steps

- This fits with the idea of snacking and doing everything in moderation, which I believe is a healthy approach to life.

Stand Snack

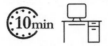

This is the simplest hack I want you to do right now, as you read this – stand up! Just do it. Get out of your chair and stand. Congratulations – just that one action is a step towards a healthier lifestyle and feeling good.

How do you feel, standing up reading this? The average adult spends 10 hours a day on their bottom, and a sedentary lifestyle increases your risk of type 2 diabetes, heart disease, cancers, general ageing and actually increases the risk of death from all causes.

Method

This is not a swap for exercise snacking but it's a reminder to get up, especially if you're a desk-based worker. It's so common to hear of people suffering from back pain due to sitting for too long.

Set a timer to remind you to stand up for a certain number of minutes every hour.

Benefits

- Helps your metabolism
- Engages your muscles
- Loads your bones

- Helps control your blood sugar levels
- Improves your posture
- Can reduce back pain and tech neck issues
- Improves your psychological health
- Burns more calories than sitting
- Can lead to significant health benefits over time, including cardiovascular and musculoskeletal benefits

Next steps

- I'm not saying stand all day, especially as standing for eight hours straight can cause tightness in the calves, hamstrings and lower back, as well as the ankles, knees and hips. I simply recommend changing positions often.
- You may find that some tasks are easier to do when you're seated. Plan your time around which jobs you do better when standing or sitting.

Top tips

- Try a standing desk versus a sitting desk.
- Stand up when you take a phone call, or set a timer for the number of standing minutes per hour.
- Consider having a stand up-style meeting instead of sitting.
- Add in some simple heel raises (great at lowering blood sugar levels after meals too).

Stand whenever you can

Just the simple act of standing gets your body systems functioning, helps your metabolism, engages your muscles, loads your bones, helps control your blood sugar levels, improves your posture and improves your psychological health. Standing can even build muscle tone. Not only do certain muscles actively engage when moving from seating to standing, they must stay engaged to keep you upright.

Replacing a few hours of sitting with standing can lead to significant health benefits over time.

This fact may intrigue you (though you know I'm not an advocate of calorie counting): when you stand, you burn anywhere from 100 to 200 calories an hour. It all depends on your sex, age, height and weight. Sitting, by comparison, only burns 60 to 130 calories an hour. Think about how fast that adds up. You could burn anywhere from 120 to 210 more calories just by swapping 3 hours of sitting for standing. While this may not help you lose a significant amount of weight, it can certainly help you maintain your current weight and reduce certain health risks.

So my message here is simple – please sit less. You can substitute sitting with at least standing up, but preferably add in other activities and try exercise snacking.

Food hacks

I could write a whole book about food. But firstly, I'm not a nutritionist, and this book is focused on exercise and taking positive steps towards feeling good. Food and fitness go hand in hand, and I know it's an area that women ask me about all the time. So here is a short section on my recommendations, plus some top tips.

Food plays such an important role throughout our life stages, but especially in midlife. Through the peri/menopause the focus should be on nourishing and caring for our bodies, not restricting or depriving them. As we get older, maintaining our usual weight can become more difficult, especially as we transition to menopause. Being careful about what we consume, our portion sizes, and doing more physical activity can all help prevent weight gain and maintain a healthy weight. Leading an active lifestyle is key, and the focus of this book is boosting well-being through my exercise and lifestyle snacks, but healthy eating and nutritious food plays such an important role too. Fitness and food work together; we need healthy food to fuel our workouts and balance our hormones. You'll also find that as you get into exercise snacking and embark on your Feel Good journey, you're more likely to make healthier and better food choices.

Exercise is like a free anti-inflammatory compound that soothes and calms everything in the body. It can satisfy cravings, aiding hunger control, and can help with satiation. As we know, weight gain – especially around the belly and abdomen area – is very common (more about this on page 12). Contributors to this so-called 'menopot' include hormonal changes (as oestrogen levels decline), age-related loss of muscle tissue, and lifestyle factors such as lack of exercise, sleep and poor diet. What we eat is even more important at this stage, and we can really take control of this. By eating to nourish your body during the menopause, you will help relieve your symptoms, reduce the risk of chronic illness and future-proof your health too.

As I said in the introduction, my mum has been pivotal in my personal approach to food and nutrition. Her philosophy has always been, 'You are what you eat, food is medicine, and you should feel good with food.' Food has always played a big part in my mental well-being, and I've never been one to skip a meal as my blood sugar levels tended to plunge when I was younger. Even now, I still get 'hangry'!

My approach is to view food as nutrition (I don't like using the word 'diet') – nutrition to fuel the body and mind. Good food makes me feel good! The Feel Good approach to nutrition is all about flexible eating and giving you the power to create your personal nutrition plan so that it is healthy, realistic and sustainable. I am not about hardcore, strict diets or fad diets – which can be hard to sustain and can cause the recurring cycle of yo-yo dieting and weight loss. There is no 'Feel Good Diet', just sensible principles to focus on when building the best possible nutrition to work around your lifestyle, goals and needs – an approach that makes you feel good and doesn't put additional stress on the body. It is about you making changes, one small but powerful habit at a time, to make sustainable lifestyle choices. Just like exercise snacks, little changes are so powerful.

I love travelling, trying new foods, new flavours and new recipes. I am vegetarian but have never felt restricted or like I'm missing out, even growing up when there was less culinary awareness. Now vegetarianism has become so popular and there is so much more variety and choice. Interestingly, I have never experienced a hot flush. A new study actually suggests that a low-fat, plant-based diet rich in soy is as effective as hormone replacement therapy (HRT) for reducing hot flushes, so maybe this is why.

Top tips to help you feel good with food

I'm going to give you a top-line summary of what I believe in. I like to focus on education and nourishment rather than restriction. I am not a nutritionist, but here are some of my top Feel Good food tips.

- **Home-cooked, whole, less processed foods are best.** I always recommend eating lots of fruit, vegetables, legumes (lentils, chickpeas, peas and beans), wholegrains, unsaturated fats (from olive oil, nuts and seeds), moderate dairy, lots of herbs and spices, less meat and few processed foods. The Mediterranean way of eating is always a good starting point and benchmark. It's low in sugar, high in fibre, and contains few or no processed foods, and is great for your gut microbiome.
- **Eat the rainbow! Feed the gut with diversity.** Remember to eat a diverse range of different colours so they are packed with vitamins, minerals, fibre and plant nutrients like antioxidants and polyphenols. Professor Tim Spector encourages us to try to eat 30 different plants a week (this includes nuts and herbs). If you do, the happier and more diverse your gut microbiome will be. The microbiome is like a garden with trillions of bacteria and microbes that live in your gut. They influence many aspects of your health, including your immune system, and they help digest the food you eat and may even play a part in keeping your bones strong. Similarly, fermented foods help keep your gut happy, so include

foods such as kefir, live yogurt, miso, kimchi, sauerkraut, kombucha and pickles.

- **Add protein to each meal for peri/menopause power.** It provides the building blocks for every cell in your body (including your muscles, bones, DNA, hormones, skin and nails). Try to add protein to every single meal – this will help balance your blood glucose/sugar levels, build lean muscle mass and support your strength/resistance training. I find it helps keep me feeling satiated, full and less likely to binge. I would aim for at least 1.2 grams of protein per kilogram of bodyweight per day during peri/menopause. I visualize this as a palm-sized portion at every meal (for example, 3 eggs, half a block of tofu/tempeh, half a cup of lentils, quinoa or edamame beans, or a pot of Greek yogurt). Starting the day with a protein-rich breakfast can help you keep your blood sugar levels steady and avoid those spikes which may affect your mood, energy and sleep. I drink a vegan protein shake daily as it's convenient and quick, especially when I'm pushed for time or on the go.

- **Don't cut out carbs.** Cutting out complex carbohydrates can exacerbate common peri/menopausal symptoms like bloating, headaches, irritability, fatigue, constipation, cholesterol issues, sugar cravings, increased insulin resistance, brain fog and mood swings. Replace refined simple carbs with complex carbohydrates. For example, go from white pasta/bread/flour to wholegrain brown options; or go from white potatoes to sweet potatoes; from cereal to oats/porridge or homemade granola. You can reduce your carbs, for sure, but I don't agree with cutting them out completely.

- **Don't count calories.** I believe in being aware of what I put in my body and nourishing it. For example, keeping a food diary or logging your food choices for a week is always a useful eye opener to help you get on track, and it will help you plan your meals for the week.

- **Plan meals ahead.** Write a menu, shop accordingly and keep healthy snacks within reach. Having a menu really helps in a family. Everyone knows what you're eating that week, and it takes a lot of stress and squabbles away. I have never given my clients prescribed meal plans, for the simple reason that I don't believe they work (although I get DMs nearly every day asking for these). A diet plan is not empowering; it takes you away from your own decision-making process – which you need for long-term success. Fitness coaches and personal trainers are not qualified to create specific meal plans for their clients. Instead of restrictive meal plans, I want to empower you to take charge of your own nutrition in a way that works for you – and feel good in the process.

- **Time-restricted eating (TRE).** This is one of the few eating patterns that doesn't have any complicated rules or regulations to remember and allows you to enjoy all your favourite foods, provided you fit all of your meals into an allotted time slot. It offers many possible health benefits, ranging from increased longevity to weight loss, improved blood sugar control and cutting the risk of type 2 diabetes, and improved sleep. It is a form of intermittent fasting and is known as 16:8 (fasting 16 hours and eating within 8) or 14:10 (fasting 14 hours, eating within 10). It basically means having a slightly later breakfast and earlier evening meal (so no late-night snacks), which can lead to some weight loss. In my midlife, I've naturally shifted my breakfast to later (I usually eat at around 11 a.m.) but I have a black coffee at 9.30 a.m. I try to stop eating by 7/8 p.m. and it seems to work for me most days.

(Though I'm not regimental about it, but I at least try to give my gut a rest from food and fast overnight for around 12–16 hours.) I think one of the biggest benefits for us women is that TRE can improve our sleep. If you're eating until late in the night, and even up to bedtime, your blood sugar levels may be elevated all night, so your body has to focus on digestion rather than vital rest and repair. We know how important sleep is (see 'Why is sleep so important?' on page 314). Chronic disruption to your circadian rhythm can lead to weight gain, inflammation, increased rates of blood pressure and disease. If you sleep better, you feel more rested the next day and in a better mental and physical state, so you're more likely to want to exercise too. TRE may not suit everyone but it's worth giving it a go.

- **Increase fibre.** This will reduce common symptoms like constipation, bloating, weight gain, sore breasts, and will help you feel full. Fibre-rich foods include vegetables, whole fruits, peas, beans, chickpeas, oats, wholegrains, nuts and flaxseeds. Build up to 30 grams of fibre per day.

- **Cut down on excess sugar.** Avoid refined sugars (like sweets, cakes and sugary drinks). Sugar can cause unnecessary heightened peri/menopausal symptoms, including mood swings, anxiety and irritability from the sugar highs and lows.

- **Reduce salt.** Avoid processed food such as ready-made meals, cooking sauces and salty snacks. Cooking from scratch means you can season and flavour food using different herbs and spices, which contain powerful nutritional benefits.

- **Eat a heart-healthy diet.** Menopause can increase the risk of developing heart disease. Eating a heart-healthy diet can help to reduce levels of cholesterol, and also lower blood pressure. Some simple hacks include:

- ° switching from saturated to unsaturated fats by cutting down on fatty meats
- ° switching to oils and spreads that are low in saturates
- ° grilling rather than frying your food.

Healthy fats include avocados, olive oil, nuts and seeds.

- **Get more plants on your plate.** Aim for half your plate to be made up of vegetables, salad, greens, pulses and beans. Green vegetables are rich in fibre, magnesium and folic acid and can help balance out your hormones and even relieve some symptoms.

- **Boost your calcium intake.** From around the age of thirty-five, we slowly lose calcium from our bones, and losing oestrogen during menopause increases this rate of loss, which can in turn increase the risk of osteoporosis. Calcium is therefore a core component that keeps our bones strong as we age, plus it can help improve meno-pausal symptoms. It can be found in cheese, yogurt, nuts and seeds, soyabeans and vegetables like broccoli.

- **Eat more soya.** Phytoestrogens derived from plants are very similar to human oestrogen, and can be useful when oestrogen levels decline during peri/menopause. They may help reduce symptoms like hot flushes. (Two servings of soya a day have been shown to reduce hot flushes to varying degrees in women.) I incorporate soya regularly through tofu, soyabeans, edamame beans, linseeds and soya milk/yogurts.

- **Adopt a low GI diet.** This can help regulate blood sugar levels. Eating foods that are slow energy release will cause a slow rise in blood sugar as opposed to a sudden one. Examples are complex carbohydrates like wholegrain bread, brown rice, pulses, beans, sweet potatoes and salad or greens.

- **Reduce caffeine and alcohol while staying hydrated with water.** This can help reduce peri/menopausal symptoms such as anxiety, poor sleep, bladder problems, UTIs, bloating, constipation, brain fog, headaches, skin issues, and can help boost your mood.

I try to get as many vitamins and minerals as possible via my food, and there's no substitute for a healthy, varied diet. But as oestrogen levels fall and hormones fluctuate, it's worth optimizing your health by making sure you get enough of the following key vitamins and minerals, perhaps with a good quality supplement.

- **Vitamin D**: This is one I have to supplement all year round (as a woman of colour). It is recommended if you live in a country with little sunshine, like the UK, as it's made by the skin's response to sunlight. It can also be found in foods like oily fish, fortified cereals and plant milks, plus some mushrooms and eggs.
- **B vitamins**: These are important in midlife, and low levels are linked to depression, low mood, low energy and irritability. Boosting them via foods like legumes, nuts, leafy vegetables and cereals can help with symptoms too.
- **Magnesium**: It can help with sleep, joint aches and pains, stress, headaches and anxiety.
- **Omega-3**: It can help alleviate hot flushes and keep your heart, brain and blood vessels healthy. Aim for 2 servings of oily fish a week. Or if you're vegetarian/vegan, opt for an algae-based supplement (as sources like nuts and seeds contain the inactive form of Omega-3 called ALA, which the body has to convert into the active forms DHA and EPA).

- **Probiotics and prebiotics**: These can be helpful for good gut health.
- **Iron**: This can be low, especially if your menstrual cycle is erratic during peri/menopause. It's best to get a blood test to check your levels.

Most importantly, remember that eating food is one of life's biggest pleasures!

Putting It into Action

I hope this book provides you with an empowering toolkit to sprinkle some Feel Good snacks regularly into your day, knowing that by just doing small bite-size amounts it can really help your health. By turning your exercise into a snack it will help you move more and sit less, improve your metabolic health and lower your disease risk, help alleviate some of the common menopausal symptoms, and future-proof yourself for longevity.

I truly believe the holistic approach of combining exercise snacks with the mind, self-care and lifestyle snacks will help you Feel Good for Life. I want you to reframe the way you think of exercise and lifestyle, to take control and start making quick and easy wins to fit into your time-pressurized life, which are sustainable in the long term too.

These methods have really helped me manage my perimenopausal symptoms, have kept me sane through life's challenges, and given me the strength and confidence to start a new career. I hope this inspires you, knowing that we can thrive through this period.

Every day I hear someone telling me how my snacks have helped them. They work! I can't wait for you to try them, share them, tag me and send me your feedback @feelgoodwithlavina.

Treat it as a pick 'n' mix, give different snacks a go. You can choose them based on the time you have available (1/3/5/10 minutes); or go by your symptoms/mood; or choose an area you'd like to focus on. There are menus at the back of the book, to make it easy for you to select which snacks you want to indulge in.

My Feel Good approach is totally flexible. There is no right or wrong. The methods in this book are all tried and tested and scientifically backed. Start off small, and of course feel free to stack some snacks (to make a meal of it). Snack your way up to 11 minutes a day! Doing activities that you enjoy, and that are easy to include in your weekly routine, is an excellent way to become more active and enjoy better health.

I want you to gain confidence, knowing that it all adds up – even a small amount of activity is better than none when it comes to improving health. *Any amount of physical activity, no matter how small, is better than none at all!* Adding up these bite-size portions to get just 11 minutes of exercise each day can have major, positive benefits on your health and longevity.

Just make a start! I want this book to tempt you to taste a variety of snacks, and as you enjoy them you will hopefully keep indulging and coming back for more. These are the only snacks I'd like you to keep nibbling, even binge on, and ideally get addicted to.

I hope the snacks you enjoy become a habit and part of your everyday lifestyle. Share them with your friends and family. Take the snacks into your workplace, your girls' get-togethers, your communities – show them, inspire them. Do the snacks when you're out and about, as they can be done anywhere. Enjoy your Feel Good Fix! Make others smile, make them curious, and give them a taste of the Feel Good snacking toolkit.

I want this book to help women of all ages, from young to old, whatever your race, background, location or lifestyle. I want these free methods to encourage you to start snacking and reap the rewards. I want women of all ages to think about living healthy lives, and take measures to be as independent and happy and disease free as they can be. I want younger women and girls to be positively prepared and equipped to look forward to what's to come, and invest in their health from a young age. I want menopausal women to know that there are lots of solutions that are going to help them embrace this part of their lives.

You are not alone, we are all different, and we can all feel good. Midlife is the perfect window of opportunity for making lifestyle changes to future-proof our health. As we get older I want us to keep strong, and keep investing in our bodies and minds. I want us to use the latest science – and this book – to Feel Good for as long as possible.

I'd love you to move well, eat well, sleep well, recover well, socialize well, work well and practise self-care and stress management – to Feel Good now and in the future.

Let's pass this book on to all the women we know, of all generations.

Let's Feel Good.

It's really never too late to start. Go for it! Pick 'n' mix to get your fix!

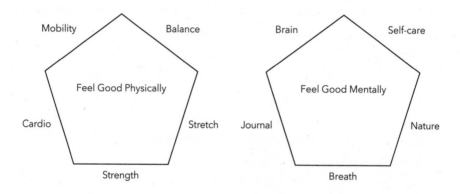

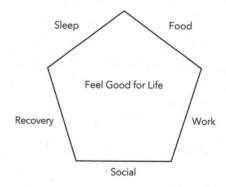

Mood menus

Here are some snacking suggestions based on your mood. Pick 'n' mix and make your own meal.

Low mood

Feel Good Hug Snack ⏱1min 🧘 *80*
Mindful Minute 5.5 Breath Snack ⏱1min 🧘 *273*
Mindful Minute Box Breath Snack ⏱1min 🧘 *279*
Mindful Minute 4-6 Breath Snack ⏱1min 🧘 *283*
Dose of Vitamin G Snack ⏱1min 📖 *285*
HIIT Snack ⏱1min ⏱5min ⏱10min 🤸 *97*
End of Day Stretch Snack ⏱1min ⏱5min ⏱10min 🧘 *92*
Wake-Up Stretch Snack ⏱3min 🧘 *127*
Gentle Seated Hormones Snack ⏱3min 🏋 *143*
Daily Wake-Up Snack ⏱5min 🧘 *154*
Feel Good Walk Snack ⏱10min 🧍🌳 *207*
Sunshine Snack ⏱10min 🌳 *305*
Heat Snack ⏱10min 🛌 *341*

Anxious and overwhelmed

Daily Affirmation Snack ⏱1min 📖 *277*
Self-care nibbles ⏱1min ⏱3min ⏱5min ⏱10min *269*
Fitness Salutation Snack ⏱3min 🧘 *124*
Yoga Balance Snack ⏱3min 🧍 *140*

Alternate Nostril Breathing Snack ⏱3min ⏱5min 🧘 289
Write Away Your Worries Snack ⏱5min 📖 293
Bird Snack ⏱5min 🌳 300
Desk Stretch Snack ⏱5min 🤸 160
Full Body Strength Snack ⏱5min ⏱10min 🏋 172
Social Media Snack ⏱10min 📱 346

Stressed

Feel Good Finish Snack ⏱1min 🤸 82
Mindful Minute Box Breath Snack ⏱1min 🧘 279
Smiling Snack ⏱1min ☀ 281
Cold Water Snack ⏱1min 🛌 338
Wake-Up Stretch Snack ⏱3min 🤸 127
Happy Hip Snack ⏱3min 🤸 130
Superbrain Snack ⏱3min ☀ 287
Tree Snack ⏱5min 🌳 295
Bird Snack ⏱5min 🌳 300
Feel Good Walk Snack ⏱10min 🚶 🌳 207

Unproductive

Stair Snack ⏱1min 🚶 106
Cold Water Snack ⏱1min 🛌 338
Dose of Vitamin G Snack ⏱1min 📖 285
Work nibbles ⏱1min ⏱3min ⏱5min ⏱10min 336
HIIT Snack ⏱1min ⏱5min ⏱10min 🚶 97
Superbrain Snack ⏱3min ☀ 287
Fitness Salutation Snack ⏱3min 🤸 124
Yoga Balance Snack ⏱3min 🧍 140
3 Goals for the Day Snack ⏱3min 📖 292

Full Body Strength Snack 🕔5min 🕙10min 🏋 *172*
Feel Good Walk Snack 🕙10min 🚶 🌳 *207*

Low energy

Cold Water Snack 🕐1min 🛌 *338*
Sprint Snack 🕐1min 🏃 *90*
Stair Snack 🕐1min 🏃 *106*
Happy Jar Snack 🕐1min 📖 *275*
HIIT Snack 🕐1min 🕔5min 🕙10min 🏃 *97*
Wake-Up Stretch Snack 🕒3min 🧘 *127*
3 Goals for the Day Snack 🕒3min 📖 *292*
Superbrain Snack 🕒3min ☀ *287*
Ad Break Snack 🕒3min 🏋 *150*
Tree Snack 🕔5min 🌳 *295*
Train the Brain Snack 🕙10min ☀ *301*
Heat Snack 🕙10min 🛌 *341*

Tired

Perfect for a restorative / calming Self-care Sunday

Pelvic Floor Snack 🕐1min 🏋 *88*
Cold Water Snack 🕐1min 🛌 *338*
Sleep tips 🕐1min 🕒3min 🕔5min 🕙10min *315*
Recovery nibbles 🕐1min 🕒3min 🕔5min 🕙10min *318*
Self-care nibbles 🕐1min 🕒3min 🕔5min 🕙10min *269*
Wake-Up Stretch Snack 🕒3min 🧘 *127*
Desk/Sofa Snack 🕔5min 🧘 *157*
Daily Wake-Up Snack 🕔5min 🧘 *154*
Cardio Seated Snack 🕔5min 🏃 *185*

Seated Strength Snack (5min) 🏋️ *188*
Seated Stretch Snack (5) 🧘 *192*
Grounding Snack (5min) 🌳 *298*
Bed Stretch Snack (10min) 🧘 *241*
Nap Snack (10) 🛌 *344*

Sitting too long

Desk Reset Snack (1min) 🧘 *76*
Tech Neck Stretch Snack (1min) 🧘 *78*
Shoulder Floss Snack (1min) 🧘 *84*
Best Back Stretch Snack (1min) 🧘 *104*
Move after meals (1min) (3min) (5min) (10min) *203*
Work nibbles (1min) (3min) (5min) (10min) *336*
HIIT Snack (1min) (5min) (10min) 🏃 *97*
Happy Hip Snack (3min) 🧘 *130*
Ad Break Snack (3min) 🏋️ *150*
Desk/Sofa Snack (5min) 🧘 *157*
Desk Stretch Snack (5min) 🧘 *160*
Full Body Mobility Snack (10min) 🧘 *198*
Back Snack (10min) 🏋️ *217*
TLC Back Snack (10min) 🧘 *194*
Indoor Step Snack (10min) 🏃 *215*
Stand Snack (10min) 🖥️ *349*

Feeling bloated

Stair Snack (1min) 🚶 *106*
Cold Water Snack (1min) 🛌 *338*
Mindful Minute 5.5 Breath Snack (1min) 🧘 *273*

Useful resources

Alzheimer's Society: www.alzheimers.org.uk/feelgood
Balance: www.balance-menopause.com
British Association for Counselling and Psychotherapy: www.bacp.co.uk
British Menopause Society: thebms.org.uk
Daisy Network: www.daisynetwork.org
Diabetes UK: www.diabetes.org.uk
Eve Appeal: eveappeal.org.uk
Exercise for Sanity, not Vanity®: TED talk by Lavina Mehta MBE at www.youtube.com/watch?v=BrRrT6FSHNO
Feel Good workouts: www.youtube.com/feelgoodwithlavina
Henpicked: henpicked.net
Menopause Charity: www.the menopausecharity.org
Menopause in the Workplace: menopauseintheworkplace.co.uk
Menopause Mandate: www.menopausemandate.com
Mind: www.mind.org.uk
NHS women's health: www.nhs.uk/womens-health
Samaritans: www.samaritans.org. Phone 116 123 for free
Shout 85258: giveusashout.org/get-help/resources
Wellbeing of Women: www.wellbeingofwomen.org.uk
Women's Aid: womensaid.org.uk
Women's Health Concern: womens-health-concern.org

Follow me on socials @feelgoodwithlavina
Find all references and notes for this book on https://feelgoodwithlavina.com/thefeelgoodfix

Acknowledgements

Where do I start? The biggest thanks go to everyone who has used or shared my workouts, as this has given me the most satisfaction, motivation and purpose to continue my mission, to help as many people as I possibly can to Feel Good! This book was a bucket list goal I added in 2020 after receiving my MBE – one that I never actually thought would happen. I have thoroughly enjoyed writing it and feel like the words have just come quite effortlessly from my mind to the page, and I hope you feel like I'm actually speaking to you. Every step of this surreal journey over the last few years has been incredible, and I'm blessed to have met and worked with some amazing people.

I know I have two guardian angels above, who shower me with their blessings: my Ba, my late grandmother Kasturben Shah, and Papa, my late father-in-law (who I have felt smiling next to me in my live workouts and interviews).

I'm grateful to my whole family. My parents – my dad, Kishore Shah, and my mum, Kumud Shah – my father-in-law, Mahendra Mehta, and my mother-in-law, Nisha Mehta. My brother, Kunal, and his wife, Jenifer, my sisters-in-law, Deepa and Chandni, and their partners, my nephews and nieces, and extended family, you all mean the world to me.

My mum has always been my inspiration, as she found her love of food at a similar point in life, when me and my brother got into secondary school, and she became an author – which I have always admired – with her books serving as her legacy forever, and the creator of the Feel Good brand! She continues to be my biggest cheerleader and best friend. She has called me after every single live, every radio/TV/press appearance and article, after every Friday Feel Good workout (often starring as my fitness buddy) and has helped me keep going with her unconditional love, encouragement, support and delicious food. Her passion, positivity and zest for life are how I aspire to live too. Thank you, Mum, for everything!

My three boys, Sai, Saj and Sahil – it's such a privilege and the biggest blessing to be your mum. Thank you for letting me follow my passion and encouraging me on this unplanned journey. You always give me the best (honest) advice, love and support, and I'm so, *so* proud of the incredible young men you have become. I love you to infinity and beyond! And, of course, our pup Bailey for being my Feel Good Walks buddy! The walks have been like a lifeline and green therapy for me – giving me time to boost my energy and focus when juggling life alongside this writing process, keeping me sane and sparking creative juices.

Thank you to my dearest husband, Menal – not only is it quite unheard of, being a PT as a South Asian woman in her forties, but especially being married and a mum! Never once have you stopped me – the opposite, you've encouraged me with every crazy idea of mine. From you and Sahil going live with me twice a day in the pandemic, to coming on to Instagram to talk about the menopause. You and the boys have seen me spend long hours, battling with tech, researching and writing this book, and I honestly wouldn't have been able to do any of it without you. You're my rock, my confidant, my best friend.

My dearest mother-in-law, without whom none of my chair workouts would have made such a huge impact on the lives of so many elderly people around the world. My Nisha, my fellow Shah girl! Who would have thought we'd become fitness buddies and feature on TV together? Thank you so much for being by my side all the way and helping so many. Your support, strength, love and prayers mean the world to me, and I'm so lucky to have you, Mummy.

Giving back via my workouts and charity work has truly been the greatest gift. A special thanks to the charities and organizations I support – as an ambassador for Diabetes UK, Alzheimer's Society, Wellbeing of Women and a patron for Menopause Mandate. I love being able to help raise awareness, vital funds and improve so many people's health. I know that together we can do amazing things to help even more people.

I want to thank lovely Gillian Joseph from Sky News who first interviewed me about Exercise Snacking on Christmas Day 2019. I'd been banging on about it, and knew in my gut I was on to something, but this was the first step in me sharing my ideas and going mainstream.

Special thanks to my Feel Good team of ladies who I've had the privilege of training in-person and virtually, and so many of you are now my dear friends.

In addition, my weekly Feel Good Workout Zoom and YouTube participants and care home residents – seeing you work out with me from home in your seventies, eighties and nineties inspires me and motivates others more than you can imagine. It has fuelled my passion even more.

Big thank you to all the communities I streamed workouts for in the pandemic, like Oshwal, Navnat, Luhana, BAPs Neasden Temple and Mahavir Foundation. Your platforms have helped me get the South Asian communities to understand the importance of movement for our health, and break so many barriers to exercise. Special thanks to Nemish, Ashish and Kaushik uncle. Thanks to all the journalists, TV, radio and press presenters, producers and social platforms that have helped me amplify my mission and messages.

My list of friends is long, and apologies if I have forgotten anyone. My closest tribe – who I know I can call anytime and you'll always be there for me, I love and appreciate you ladies always – Jeni, Meenal, Komal, Jayshree, Vandna, Heeral, Alpa, Ekta, Davita, Leena, Amiee, Shweta, Sairha and Seema.

My third set of parents, Naresh and Bhavna Bhuva, my uni friends, my corporate work colleagues, my school mum friends, my men-on-pause neighbours gang, to all my walking buddies – you have all been a part of my life and journey (this is not an exhaustive list!).

My Menopause Mandate family, fellow patrons and friends – Davina McCall, Michelle Griffith Robinson, Cherry Healey, Lisa Snowdon, Carol Vorderman, Penny Lancaster, Carolyn Harris, Laura Biggs, Melissa Robertson. Huge thanks to the founders, Mariella Frostrup and Alice Smellie, for getting me involved after I stood up declaring my perimenopause at their book launch in April 2022. I love the impact and work we all do together.

I have made some recent but close friendships on social media, people I feel like I've known all my life – Dr Nighat Arif, Michelle and Cherry, Aziza, Sooj, to name a few. So many meno warriors and campaigners who are so passionate to drive change for women's health – I appreciate you, let's keep going!

I'm so lucky to have spoken to some inspiring authors who gave me their advice when my book proposal (unimaginably) went to a bidding auction – Dr Rangan Chattergee, Dr Ayan Panja, Dr Julie, Simon Alexander Ong – and the support and encouragement in my journey from experts like Professor Tim Spector, Louise Newson, Lorraine Candy, Rosie Nixon and Mo Gawdat. Rangan, I'll never forget our first interaction during the Covid pandemic, onstage with you in a Clubhouse room, when you said, 'Lavina, all doctors should be prescribing your workouts.' This is still my goal!

My YouTube Health buddies – and a special mention to Dr Vishaal Virani and Alison Lomax MD.

Everyone who has 'exercise snacked' with me at events, from unimaginable places like the Houses of Parliament and outside Number 10, to the workplaces and companies I have been able to do special events and talks for. Snacking with you has brought me so much joy!

To everyone who has followed and supported my journey and ideas on social media – every like, every comment, every DM and feedback has added so much value and fuelled my purpose. You have helped me pursue my passion and share my message with more people than I ever thought imaginable.

Finally, the team that has made this actually happen – turning my dream into a reality. This book is such a dream come true! It was fate, how I met my amazing literary agent Therese Coen, who just got me and the book the minute we met. It's such an honour to be with my dream publishing house, Penguin – the books I grew up reading. None of this would be possible without the dream team at Penguin Life. To my incredible editor, Emily, heartfelt thanks for all your guidance, input, help and vision – I honestly couldn't have asked for anyone better, you understand me and how I imagined this book. I have loved the publishing and writing process so much, thanks to Thérèse and Emily. To my copy editor, Shân, and the whole team at Penguin, to name a few – Preena Gadher, Julia Murday, Martina O'Sullivan, Annie Moore, Ruth Johnstone, Ellie Smith, Sara Granger, Fran Monteiro. I'll never forget the words they told me at my signing celebration: that when they read my proposal it was like a breath of fresh air and they just had to publish it. Thank you for believing in me and for bringing it to life.

Every word in this book comes from my heart, and I truly hope you feel that. So I thank you, the reader, and I really hope you experience and enjoy The Feel Good Fix!

Special thanks to Will Carne for brilliantly filming and editing the videos (the most clips he's ever filmed in two days!). Having QR codes was my husband's brainwave, and I love how it transforms publishing, from traditional fitness workout photos and illustrations, to me actually guiding you as a companion to this book.